SMART BLOOD SUGAR

The Complete System to
Naturally Balance Blood Sugar
and Prevent or Reverse Diabetes
. . . Without Drugs!

Second Edition

Dr. Marlene Merritt, DOM, MS Nutrition

Disclaimer

This book offers health, medical, fitness, and nutritional information for educational purposes only. This information has not been evaluated by the FDA and is not intended to treat, diagnose, cure, or prevent any disease. You should not rely on this information as a substitute or a replacement for professional medical advice, diagnosis, or treatment.

You should, however, seek the advice of your healthcare provider before undertaking any treatment or if you have any concerns or questions about your health. Do not disregard, avoid, or delay obtaining medical or health-related advice from your healthcare professional because of something you may have read in this book. Nothing stated here is intended to be, and must not be taken to be, the practice of medical, nutritional, physiological, or any professional care.

Primal Health, LP and its officers, directors, and trainers disclaim any warranties (expressed or implied), of merchantability, or fitness for any particular purpose, and shall in no event be held liable to any party for any direct, indirect, punitive, special, incidental or other consequential damages arising directly or indirectly from any use of this material, which provided "as is," and without warranties.

Images used under license from Shutterstock.com.

Primal Health, LP
710 Century Parkway
Allen, TX 75013

Printed in the United States of America

First Printing, 2015
Second Printing, 2017

TABLE OF CONTENTS

EDITOR'S PREFACE

After only two short years in circulation, it is an absolute delight to be publishing a second edition of *Smart Blood Sugar*. Tens of thousands of people have looked to Dr. Marlene Merritt's book in hopes of finding a way out of the medical industry's grip, and they have found that there absolutely is a way to escape the shadow of diabetes.

As this book is making its rounds across the world, it has garnered much attention and a lot of feedback from its readers—and all of us at Primal Health were listening. The Second Edition we present you with today is a complete, top-to-bottom reworking of this bestselling book. Not only has it been updated to include more recent research on the subject of diabetes, but we have expanded upon several topics to specifically address the feedback received from its past readers. Our hope is that those to come will find an even more complete discussion of how to balance their blood sugar safely and naturally.

With a new look and feel, readers will find this book to be visually engaging (and easy on the eyes)! Sections have been added to address calorie consumption, diabetes myths, and the growing list of serious conditions related to blood sugar imbalance. Additionally, we've included extended discussions on natural solutions to our readers' health concerns.

What has not changed, however, is the wit and wisdom of the author. Dr. Merritt's work is always carried out with rigorous attention to detail, but she never lets the scientific jargon overwhelm her ability to help us understand complex ideas as simple, scientific solutions. Reading this book won't feel like a frightening trip to the doctor's office, but rather a pleasant conversation with a well-informed friend who wants you to live a longer and happier life.

So, read on, and get ready to meet the new you!

INTRODUCTION

WHY YOUR DOCTOR'S RECOMMENDATIONS ARE NOT WORKING

There could be any number of reasons why you have made the decision to read this book. Perhaps because you, or someone you love, is facing the scary reality of a pre-diabetes, or diabetes diagnosis. Or perhaps your own research on topics such as cancer, depression, fatigue, digestive issues, weight gain, and/or hormonal imbalances has led you to discover that many of these health issues are interrelated. Or maybe a family history has led to your concern of experiencing any of these issues firsthand.

Or sadly, you may be reading this because you are seeking an alternative not only to the physical effects of diabetes, but to the more recent financial hardships diabetics on insulin therapy are facing today. It's no secret that pharmaceutical companies frequently offer "new and improved" versions of the same medications (most likely with the primary goal of maintaining possession of revenue-generating, patented products). Of course, these new (non-generic) brands come with an extraordinary increase in cost—for practically the same product! As diabetes diagnoses are at an all-time high, drug companies are happy to compete for your business. For patients with medical insurance, these price increases may go relatively unnoticed. But if you are insulin-dependent and have little to no prescription coverage, you may be facing a life-threatening situation, simply because you can no longer afford your prescriptions. Understandably, you're desperate for a solution. You're not alone—I'm here to help.

In today's world, with high-tech tools at our fingertips, it's become second nature to get on the internet seeking information that gives us a clearer understanding of things. Unfortunately, the overwhelming wealth of information you find may only lead to more confusion.

Whatever your reason for picking up this book, I am so very glad you did—because I want to offer clear explanations that provide a logical understanding of how to address your health concerns. I also want to give you all the tools you need to reverse what seems to be inevitable for too many people. And furthermore, I'm going to show you how to do it *naturally* . . . without drugs.

I've had a lot of patients come into my office in Austin, Texas, who follow my recommendations, and get great results. They always ask me why their doctor didn't give them the same advice that I did, and I smile as I respond, "Good question." Part of the reason why many doctors don't give you the advice you'll see here is because for decades, the medical establishment has been married to the idea that fat is bad and carbs are good. It's hard to let go of something you've said for years and years—even when the research doesn't support it.

You'll see. Once you follow the recommendations I've laid out here and get the results you've desired, the whole thing will seem obvious to you: if you want to regulate your blood sugar, stop filling your body with sugar or things that turn into sugar.

It'll seem obvious, too, that medications can't cure someone who's still eating poorly. It's tough to put out a blaze when you keep pouring more fuel on it. But if you fill yourself with the right foods, and begin making the right lifestyle choices, those adverse health conditions can often reverse themselves—or better yet, you won't even get them in the first place!

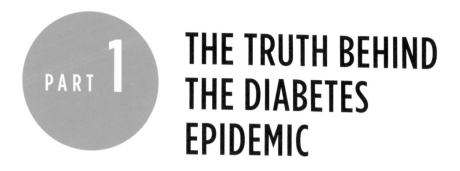

THE TRUTH BEHIND THE DIABETES EPIDEMIC

PART 1

DANGERS OF BLOOD SUGAR IMBALANCES

Blood sugar imbalances can cause dozens of different problems; from the minor but constant annoyances, to the serious and potentially fatal conditions.

Starting With the Worst

Diabetes: One out of eleven people in America have Type 2 diabetes. But amazingly, a quarter of those don't even know they have it. Even worse, more than one in three adults are pre-diabetic, and nine-tenths of those don't know it.[1] And most people don't really get the impact. High blood glucose damages blood vessels and makes the blood too thick to pass through the little capillaries in your body—the ones that supply blood to important organs like your kidneys and eyes. That's why every 24 hours, 230 diabetics lose a limb, 55 will go blind, and 120 will experience kidney failure.[2] Did you know that diabetes is the #1 cause of erectile dysfunction, and that the risk of early death is 50% higher for people with diabetes than without?

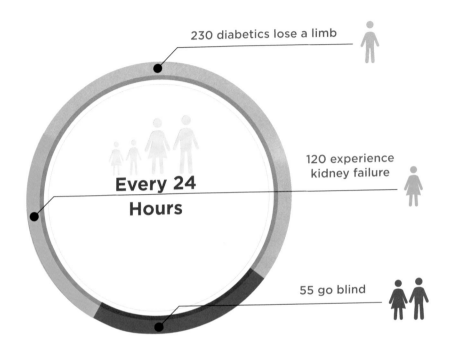

Diabetics Have a 50% Higher Risk of Early Death Compared to Non-Diabetics

230 diabetics lose a limb

Every 24 Hours

120 experience kidney failure

55 go blind

Hypertension: We're quick to think that high blood pressure is mostly caused by salt, but "the wrong white crystals" are being blamed.[3] Interestingly, if you eat too little salt, that can speed up insulin resistance![4] (We'll describe insulin resistance in more detail later.) So, if you want to manage high blood pressure, the first thing to do is stop eating processed foods and sugar!

Cardiovascular Disease and Strokes: Most people have no idea that it's actually insulin and glucose that cause you to have the small, dense Type b LDL cholesterol that causes plaques and not, (as we've been told for so many years), saturated fat.[8,9] This is because it's glucose that's vulnerable to oxidation (which causes plaques). So since high blood sugar makes the blood thicker and stickier, incidence of blood clots and strokes go way up.[10] People with diabetes, are 180% more likely to have a heart attack, 170% more likely to die of cardiovascular disease, and two and a half times as likely to have a stroke.[11]

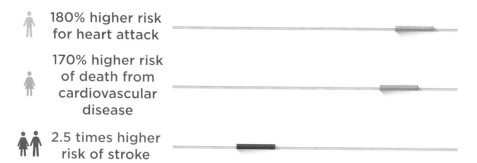

180% higher risk
for heart attack

170% higher risk
of death from
cardiovascular
disease

2.5 times higher
risk of stroke

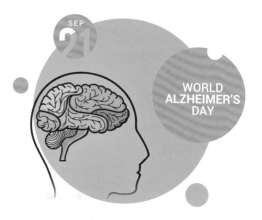

Alzheimer's Disease: Alzheimer's results from insulin resistance in the brain, which is why some researchers are starting to refer to it as Type 3 Diabetes.[12] If you're diagnosed with diabetes before the age of 65, it doubles your chances of developing Alzheimer's.[13]

Cancer: Do you know that cancer cells can only use glucose as a fuel? This is actually not new information—the researcher Otto Warburg discovered this in the 1920's, and his discovery was named the Warburg Effect. In modern cancer treatment, oncologists have used PET scans as one of their main diagnostic tools since the 1980s. The way PET scans work is by giving the patient radioactive glucose and then scanning their body to see where it went. Lewis Cantley, director of the Cancer Center at Harvard Medical School, says that up to 80% of all human cancers have glucose and insulin as instigating factors.[14] Dr. Craig Thompson, researcher and president of New York's Memorial Sloan-Kettering Cancer Research Center, believes that many pre-cancerous cells would never become malignant if it wasn't for the constant exposure to insulin and needing glucose for their metabolism.[15]

> "...many pre-cancerous cells would never become malignant if it wasn't for the constant exposure to insulin..."

Chronic Pain and Autoimmune Disorders: Both glucose and insulin are highly inflammatory, and inflammation leads to joint pain, arthritis, fibromyalgia and other chronic pain conditions and autoimmune disorders. We've had patients who've cured years of chronic pain—in just a couple of weeks—simply by cutting out sugar.

Depression and Anxiety: Both depression and anxiety are poorly affected by sugar, as insulin prevents amino acids from crossing the blood-brain barrier, prohibiting your neurotransmitters from functioning effectively. In fact, having diabetes doubles your chances of being diagnosed with depression.[16] Once people get their blood sugar under control, incidences of anxiety and panic attacks drop dramatically.

Weight Gain: Isn't it frustrating? You're eating the way they tell you to, but you can't ever seem to lose weight and keep it off for more than a few months. The reason, for most people, is that insulin prevents fat from being burned. So every time you eat a carb and release insulin into your bloodstream, you put on more weight.

Fatty Organs: It's not just your waistline that gets fat—your organs can get fat as well, inside the cells. This happens from the overload of calories and is shockingly prevalent among the overweight. We'll talk more about this later, but it's not limited to just a fatty liver—you can have a fatty heart, fatty pancreas, and even a fatty tongue!

Gas and Bloating: This might seem like a no-brainer, but your digestive system doesn't like sugar. This is because you're not the only one who uses glucose for energy—bacteria do, too, and carbs feed the wrong bacteria in your gut, causing lots of gas. This is one of the first things to change when you cut down on carbs!

Fatigue or Insomnia: Blood sugar roller coasters are just exhausting! Difficulty waking up, food comas, insomnia, and being tired all day (or at particular times of the day), are all symptoms of blood sugar imbalances. Do you ever wake up in the middle of the night and have trouble getting back to sleep? Your body may be giving you a shot of adrenalin, because it's afraid you might slip into a coma otherwise. This can be caused from the years of sugar abuse tiring out your adrenal glands. Your adrenals help to ensure that your brain stays fed, but once your blood sugar system is "broken", and your adrenals are tired out, it's hard to keep things stable at night. Improving your blood sugar solves all these problems, and you'll have better energy in just a handful of days.

Your Immune System: A blood sugar count of over 120 causes your white blood cell function to drop 75% for over four hours![17] So if you find yourself constantly getting sick, there's a good chance sugar has something to do with it.

Hormonal Problems: High blood sugar causes multiple hormone imbalances. For men, one of the most obvious is high estrogen, which produces "man boobs" and beer bellies, and both men and women experience weight gain. Estrogen is also tied to multiple cancers, including breast,[5] uterine,[6] and prostate,[7] as well as infertility. And estrogen prevents testosterone from functioning properly, leading to "low T" symptoms such as sexual dysfunction, low energy, depression, and reduced muscle mass. In some women, high blood sugar also causes high testosterone, causing female-pattern hair loss (FPHL), facial hair growth, and poly-cystic ovarian disease.

High Blood Pressure Discrimination: Age and Gender

While it's true that percentages for both men and women are almost equal when it comes to the likelihood of developing high blood pressure in their lifetimes, hormones and age are two important variables that can affect both men and women differently.

Hormonal Imbalances

When it comes to problems associated with these chemical messengers, particularly estrogen and testosterone, high blood pressure shows no gender discrimination.

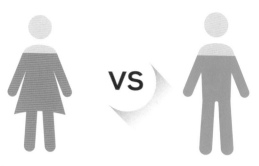

VS

Weight Gain
Breast and Uterine Cancer
Infertility
Sexual Dysfunction
Low Energy
Depression
Facial Hair Grown
Poly-cystic Ovarian Disease
Female-Pattern Hair Loss

"Man Boobs"
"Beer Belly"
Weight Gain
Prostate Cancer
Infertility
Sexual Dysfunction
Low Energy
Depression
Reduced Muscle Mass
Male-Pattern Baldness

Age Before Beauty? Not necessarily.

Comparably, there's little difference in likelihood for developing high blood pressure for men and women, on average. But once age becomes a factor, those percentages will change.

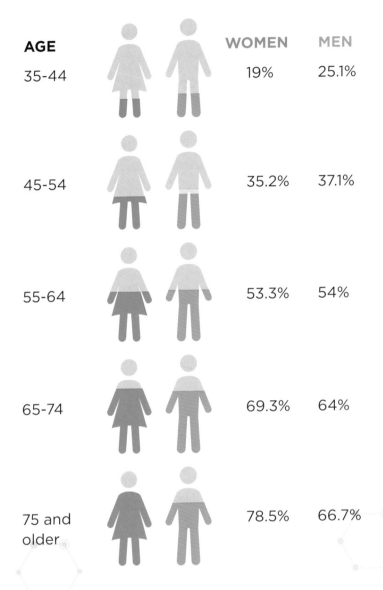

AGE			WOMEN	MEN
35-44			19%	25.1%
45-54			35.2%	37.1%
55-64			53.3%	54%
65-74			69.3%	64%
75 and older			78.5%	66.7%

Clearly, the impact here is more than just the "sugar crash" our parents talked about when we were kids. So if you want to know the truth about the diabetes epidemic what needs to be done in order to manage blood sugar, keep reading.

UNDERSTANDING BLOOD SUGAR AND INSULIN

Highs and Lows of Blood Sugar

One way of looking at blood sugar is to think about it like a campfire. When you were camping and built a fire, you might have started it with newspaper, but you didn't have someone standing there for the next two hours throwing newspaper in, did you? No, you kept the fire burning more consistently by using denser forms of fuel, like larger logs.

It's the same with blood sugar. To keep blood sugar stable (meaning, not going too high or too low), you have to feed yourself foods that aren't like newspaper on flames. When it comes to your blood sugar, you can think of a cookie like a newspaper on the flames. Yes, it will give you energy, but you'll burn right through that energy in about 30 minutes, and your fire will go out. If you have this issue, you might have realized that you have to keep yourself fed to prevent blood sugar drops, but it just doesn't work to keep feeding your flame of energy with the equivalent of newspaper.

This may come as a shock to hear at first, but the best way to keep things stable is to add fat into your diet. In fact, before insulin was discovered and used, diabetics were treated with a high-fat diet![18] You may be skeptical about this at first, but let's take look at a couple of scenarios to better understand how food choices affect blood sugar imbalances.

The Path to Insulin Resistance

One of the first things to understand about diabetes is that it doesn't happen overnight. It takes years of drinking soda, ordering dessert, getting candy bars from the vending machine, downing energy drinks for a little boost, and eating mountains of mashed potatoes, spaghetti, and popcorn to cause your system to break down. So how does this happen?

One concept to keep in mind as you read: all carbohydrates break down into sugar, which is why the terms are often used interchangeably in this book. Even carbohydrates with fiber (so-called "good carbs") will ultimately break down to glucose, an important concept that dieticians often seem to forget.

So let's start with a hypothetical, normal, healthy person. If this person eats cereal, that cereal will go into his or her stomach and through the small intestines. There, the cereal breaks down into glucose, which travels through the walls of the small intestines and into the blood. Now, this is what is called blood glucose, and it is this blood glucose that is measured on blood tests.

When glucose enters this hypothetical person's bloodstream, their body wants to process it as quickly as possible. So the pancreas releases insulin, whose job is to "carry" the glucose from the bloodstream to all the cells in the body. Since our hypothetically normal person is healthy, his system is working perfectly. His pancreas releases the precise amount of insulin it needs based on the amount of glucose in the blood.

Unfortunately, I almost never see that person in my office.

Because for most people, after years of high-carb eating, their system starts trying to "predict" how much insulin is going to be needed. You've been eating a high amount of carbs, so your body gives you a lot of insulin to deal with it. That insulin does the job it's supposed to, which is get the glucose into the cells, but the problem is that the extra insulin can also drop your blood sugar below the ideal levels.

The first organ that gets affected is your brain, because your body needs a minimum of 30% blood sugar in order for your brain to function properly. So that's when the fatigue, memory issues, concentration problems, and irritability kick in—because your brain is hungry!

Additionally, this constant imbalance of sugar causes you to crave more sugar. People keep thinking they have willpower problems, but that extra insulin is "looking" for sugar. It's not in your head, nor is it just "luck" that some people seem to have willpower—it's actually all about your physiology.

And insulin also prevents you from burning fat. Yes, you heard that right—insulin is a storage hormone, meaning it makes fat and prevents you from burning it. So every time you eat anything containing a carbohydrate, insulin is released, and that insulin prevents you from accessing your fat stores.

Most people notice that when they're hungry and their brain isn't working well, that everything gets better when they eat something. We mostly turn to simple high-carb foods like chips or crackers or energy bars, because they're cheap, easy to keep on hand, and they're addictive. Oh, and easy to metabolize. So while your brain will feel better temporarily, it has also released insulin again to deal with those carbs. This process can drop your blood sugar again, which makes you hungry again, and causes the cycle to repeat.

After doing this again, and again, and again... over a period of several years, the constant presence of insulin starts to "annoy" the insulin receptors on the cells, and some of them become resistant, meaning that they cease to function properly. Now glucose can't get into that cell, and it continues to float around your bloodstream. Your body recognizes this as a problem, so it moves the glucose out of the bloodstream by turning it into fat. It's the process of converting sugar into fat that produces triglycerides.

As time goes on, more and more tissues become resistant, your blood sugar starts to rise, and you finally pass 100 on your blood test. At this point, your doctor might tell you that you have insulin resistance or pre-diabetes; however, in reality, you've had it for years. Your body has just been desperately trying to adapt to the problem.

Many people try to make some changes at this point, but usually those changes aren't effective or comprehensive enough, as they're still consuming "good carbs" even if they cut out the simple ones. Even though the fiber in a whole grain will slow down how quickly glucose enters the bloodstream, when your system is primed for insulin, a whole grain carb will still be treated just like any other carb. And that carb still causes an overreaction of insulin, so the process continues.[19]

As blood sugar continues to rise, the only way the body can deal with it is to push the pancreas to make more and more insulin in an attempt to force the glucose into the cells. However, this process only causes the overworked pancreas to fail due to exhaustion. This is the point at which you will be diagnosed as a diabetic; your body just can't produce enough insulin anymore. As you can see, though, your blood sugar problems have been progressing for decades at this point.

The Path Towards Diabetes

Insulin resistance happens at different speeds, but for most people it often goes undetected, particularly in the early stages.

━━ **STAGE 1** ━━ Childhood, Adolescence, and Early 20's

━━ **STAGE 2** ━━ Early to Late 30's

━━ **STAGE 3** ━━ Early 40's - Late 50's

━━ **STAGE 4** ━━ 60 and Older

By the age of 65, 77% of adults are diabetic or pre-diabetic.

If we focus on this path to insulin resistance in terms of stages, we may be able to pinpoint where things started going wrong. Remember, this whole process happens at different speeds for many people—some may have been able to stave off this process a bit longer by just by getting more exercise. Yet for others, having grown up accustomed to drinking soda and typically sitting around on the couch, this process likely progressed much more rapidly. Becoming a Type 2 diabetic is not a coincidental occurrence. Most people go through the stages as we will discuss below, but as traditional MD's are not trained to catch the earlier stages, it generally goes unnoticed. As you read, you may recognize some patterns that could help pinpoint when these stages may have occurred for you:

STAGE 1: A lot of patterns start in your childhood, adolescence, and your 20's. Maybe you grew up eating dessert every night, enjoyed having cookies and milk or regularly drinking soda in your house, because it was provided for you all the time. Maybe during your high school years you binged on candy at the corner store, or bought fast food items for your lunch. Or, perhaps when you went to college or started living on your own, you ate sugar cereal for breakfast (or lunch, or dinner!) and drank soda because… well, it was there. During this phase of your life, you probably just ate what people around you ate, to some degree.

For most people, this is usually when it all started. And like them, you probably never noticed any symptoms, though some may begin gaining weight.

STAGE 2: As you entered your 30's, your pants may have begun feeling tighter, and you may have noticed that you were getting tired more easily than you used to. You could have experienced ups and downs with your energy, noticing that you felt better after you had something to eat. Did you notice having sugar cravings a lot more often? How about insomnia issues? If you're a woman, your periods may have become problematic.

STAGE 3: In your 40's and 50's—that's when everything starts to get real. You officially have an expanding waistline, which many will blame on menopause or middle age. You're tired. A LOT. You wake up at night, you sleep too lightly, and you have a hard time getting out of bed in the morning. You start compiling diagnoses—high blood pressure, high cholesterol, high triglycerides, anxiety and/or depression, thyroid issues, etc… Your life is stressful, and you might eat to feel better. You still crave sugar a lot, and you know it doesn't work for you, but you eat it anyway, in a subconscious (or conscious) attempt to feel better. You try some diets, and while they help for a little while, nothing sticks. You start to feel hopeless.

But if your doctor knows about nutrition (most don't, but there are some exceptions out there), they might start discussing sugar intake with you, but it'll be a vague sort of suggestion like, "eat less sugar," which you probably already know. You try to do that, but the sugar cravings just overcome you, and you can't stay on the wagon. This is when your doctor might mention the words "pre-diabetic."

STAGE 4: Once you've reached your 60's and older, you might be totally resigned to what's happening to your body at this point. You're overweight; the doctor mentions that you could reverse your hypertension by losing weight, but you are pretty sure you've tried everything, and nothing has worked. Your sleep has either never improved, or gotten worse. You might be on a C-Pap machine (or you should be). Your energy is in the toilet—you want to play with your grandkids, but they wear you out. In fact, everything wears you out. You may deal with a cancer diagnosis, or have the responsibility of caring for an aging parent. And don't be surprised by a fear of dementia if you notice that you're not feeling quite as sharp as you used to be—your mortality is starting to stare you in the face.

By the age of 65, 77% of adults are diabetic or pre-diabetic.[20] And that's just one issue. There is also Metabolic Syndrome

What Is Metabolic Syndrome?

The typical indicators of metabolic syndrome is having three or more of the following conditions at the same time:

- High triglycerides

- High fasting blood glucose

- Low HDL

- An expanding waistline

- High blood pressure

You are more likely to develop metabolic syndrome when you begin gaining weight, and it's associated with increased hormonal problems. And fatigue, high blood sugar, and cardiovascular problems are only compounded when digestive issues and immune/autoimmune disorders may start to appear.

Pushing the Limit

Have you ever really thought about how many times a day you actually consume sugar, or something that turns into sugar?

We eat more sugar and refined carbs in a week than people who lived 200 years ago ate in one year!

Let's say you eat cereal with fruit in the morning (all carbs and sugar). Add milk to that . . . milk has sugar in it, too (lactose). You go into the office, and grab a donut in the break room on the way to your desk (all sugar). To wash it down, you have a cup of coffee with creamer (which often has some sugar in it), and then you add a little more sugar.

At lunch, you have a turkey sandwich and chips or a piece of fruit (it all becomes sugar except for the turkey). You have a mocha latte to "pick you up" in the afternoon (all sugar except for the espresso).

For dinner, you meet your friends at your favorite Mexican restaurant, where you have a delightful margarita (sugar), chips (carbs becoming sugar) and salsa, and three fish tacos (the tortillas are carbs becoming sugar).

Wow! That's a lot of carbs and sugar in one day when you really look at it. And that really is the typical American diet. We eat more sugar and refined carbs in a week than people who lived 200 years ago ate in one year. And every time sugar shows up in your system, your body produces insulin to try to process it.

I often explain it to people this way: It's kind of like we were given a certain number of "points" for carbs in our lifetimes, and most of us have used up those points by the age of 30 or 35. The problem is that we often don't know that we're out of points until much later. By that time, though, we are well on our way to diabetes. And with kids nowadays, it's actually much sooner—adolescents are the fastest growing population of diabetics. This current generation of kids is the first one that will not live as long as their parents, primarily because of this disease.

DIAGNOSING PRE-DIABETES/ DIABETES

There are three tests that give an indication of how someone's blood sugar is doing. Most people are familiar with the "Glucose" measurement on a fasting blood test. This is the one that is most volatile and can change drastically depending on what you ate last night.

Another is the "Triglycerides" measurement, which is also an indicator of how you eat, but it assesses the breakdown of carbohydrates. When the glucose builds up in the blood, the body shunts a lot of that into fat, and your triglyceride levels increase. While it's not ALWAYS from carbohydrate intake, most frequently triglycerides over 100 mg/dl indicate higher carb intake. An ideal range is in the ballpark of 70 mg/dl.

The best test is the Hemoglobin A1c test, which is an average of your blood sugar levels over a 3 month period. Basically, if you have red blood cells floating in the sugar solution in your blood stream, they'll start to accumulate a coating of sugar (the technical term for this is "glycation"). The more sugar in your bloodstream, the thicker the coating, and this amount of thickness is what is measured in this test. At our practice, we start discussing carb intake with people when the number is 5.5% or higher. Laboratory testing designates pre-diabetes at 5.7%, and diabetes as 6.5%.

DOWNSIDE OF STANDARD MEDICAL TREATMENTS

The downside of traditional diabetes treatments is probably best explained by saying that we're trying to treat chronic illness in an acute care model. This means that we're mostly just reacting to a disease—trying to manage it with medications and symptom control—rather than actually dealing with the root problem and treating the foundational issues.

The way diabetes is often treated is a great example of this kind of treatment—both for Type 1 and Type 2. In Type 1 diabetes, called "insulin-dependent diabetes," the advice to patients is basically to match their insulin injections to what they eat. Eat a high-carb meal? Inject a little more. It's often not explained to these patients that long-term exposure to insulin (and this is also true for Type 2) causes a lot of harm. We're going to talk about that in a bit more detail in a moment.

In Type 2 diabetes, it's often not treated early enough or aggressively enough. Remember, this condition didn't develop overnight. This happened over the years leading up to the diagnosis, but most people's doctors didn't have the knowledge about what to do, diet- or lifestyle-wise, or they didn't have the time to have the conversations . . . and they often just see patients once a year, so how can they really follow up and support someone?

That's why treatment seems to lead to medication at some point. The disease progresses. People are getting worse. And without good support and knowledge, people just don't know what to do. So they fill the prescriptions they are given, and things either get better, or they don't. People either improve what they eat, or they don't. If they don't, the next medication is prescribed, or an associated disease is diagnosed with its accompanying medication, and the cycle continues.

When things progress to the point of someone needing to take insulin injections, it is because their overworked and exhausted pancreas just can't make insulin anymore. Now they're just like a Type 1 diabetic who simply had to do this their whole life.

The problem is, though, that insulin comes with some significant issues, especially long-term use of insulin. There's an increased risk of cancer,[21,22,23] and there is also an increased risk of mortality.[24] There's a significant increase in weight gain with the onset of insulin therapy—as one study showed, there can be an increase of nearly 20 pounds in only 6 months![25]

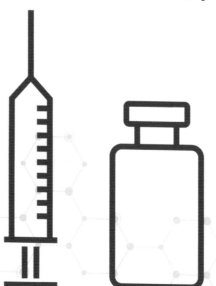

Insulin Comes With Significant Risks

- CANCER
- DEATH
- WEIGHT GAIN
- long-term increase in CARDIOVASCULAR EVENTS and SURGERIES

There's also a significant increase in cardiovascular issues, both for Type 1 and Type 2 diabetics with insulin therapy. One study saw that the weight gain mentioned above definitely also included Type 2 diabetics, but also included a long-term increase in cardiovascular risk.[26] Multiple other studies done on Type 2 diabetics saw that, compared to diabetics on other diabetic medications, the patients on insulin fared worse in cardiovascular events and surgeries.[27,28]

Once you're on insulin, it's very hard to come off of it, mainly because your pancreas has already become quite damaged (after all, that's why you went on it in the first place). It's definitely possible to no longer be insulin dependent—we've had a couple of people who radically changed their diets, taking stress off their pancreas—so the remaining cells recovered, and their insulin output increased, meaning they needed less and less insulin. But after seeing the list above, outlining the issues with insulin, being able to need less is a very big deal and absolutely a goal to shoot for. This is how we work with Type 1 diabetics as well. NO ONE needs more insulin, and the best way to manage that is by managing diet.

DIABETES MYTHS & FACTS

We have already gone over some key facts about diabetes, but there ARE some myths:

Type 1 Diabetes

MYTH: It's OKAY for you to eat carbs, as long as you take enough insulin to match it.

This is typically how many Type 1 diabetics function—some of them DO manage their carb intake, but the guidelines given to them by traditional medicine allow for far more carbs (and therefore insulin) than is healthy. The damaging effects of insulin we have just seen apply to Type 1 diabetics as well, and perhaps even more so, because they've typically been injecting insulin for far longer than Type 2 diabetics.

In fact, back in the times before insulin was invented, they managed Type 1 diabetes by putting patients on a high-fat diet—70% fat, to be exact.[29] Only 8% carbs. That diet saved many people who would have died otherwise, as this was the only way to lower blood glucose to a safe level.

We have many Type 1 diabetics in our clinic who understand this, so by modifying their diets, and reducing their carb consumption, they only have to take a little insulin. They monitor themselves closely, but many of them have been doing that successfully for years, to the surprise of their more traditional doctors!

Type 2 Diabetes

MYTH: You can't reverse Type 2 Diabetes.

This is completely incorrect. Now, it DOES depend on how long and how much damage you've done to your pancreas, because at a certain point, it is very hard to restore function. By the time someone gets a diagnosis of Type 2 diabetes, it's estimated that 50% of their pancreatic beta cells have died, and the remaining 50% are stressed and struggling.

The sooner you can take the pressure off those remaining cells, the greater your chance is to get them stronger and possibly back to normal. The thing is, many people are either told that this is impossible, or they don't want to do what it takes to get better. But since you're reading this, I'm going to assume you want to avoid all of the horrific health conditions that come with diabetes—more on how to do that in Part 2!

REAL CAUSES BEHIND THE DIABETES EPIDEMIC

When Did It All Begin?

It's actually a relatively new phenomenon, this diabetes epidemic. Up until the early 1980's, only one in seven people were obese, and it had been the same for decades. Yes, that's correct—the obesity rate had not changed substantially for years and years. However, a few big public health changes occurred in recent decades.

When Fat Became Public Enemy Number One

Starting in the 1970's, we heard time and time again that saturated fat would clog our arteries, and that to be healthy and thin, we needed to cut down on our fat intake as much as possible.

Remember the Food Pyramid?

Look at that. A tiny bit of fat at the top, and 6-11 servings of carbohydrates at the bottom.

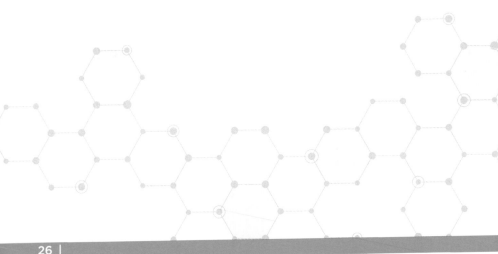

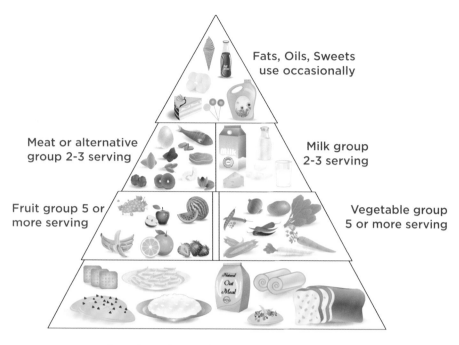

Fats, Oils, Sweets
use occasionally

Meat or alternative
group 2-3 serving

Milk group
2-3 serving

Fruit group 5 or
more serving

Vegetable group
5 or more serving

Breads and Cereals group 6-11 serving

The Deception of Healthy Recommendations

There were a few problems with this; mostly that it wasn't based on good science. The body prefers fat as a fuel. Remember our metaphor from the beginning—how fueling your body with carbohydrates is a bit like throwing newspaper on flames? Fat is the "big log," burning slowly for a long time, keeping your blood sugar stable and your brain well fed, because it doesn't break down nearly as fast. This means you feel better for longer periods of time.

And for those of you with high blood sugar, the same applies. Fats do not trigger insulin, and they don't break down into glucose. They'll keep your energy stable by giving your body an alternate source of fuel (called ketones) which is super important if you're trying to lower your blood sugar with diet.

...an entire nation changed its way of eating based on a combination of scant evidence and political economics.

This pyramid also neglected the fact that fat makes you feel full—remove it, and people are hungry most of the time. Does this sound familiar? And contrary to what might seem like common sense now (because of what we've been told over and over again), saturated fat does *not* actually clog your arteries.

You heard that right. You may have heard it a million times that butter and red meat will block your arteries and kill you, but when you actually look at the research, there are a couple of situations that got muddled up. I'll talk more about that muddling-up later, but right now it's important to note that the woman who originally came up with the Food Pyramid—a highly lauded nutritionist—recommended almost the opposite of what you see above.[30]

In her original food pyramid, grains came in at no more than two to three servings per day. She also suggested, in addition to fats we get naturally from foods, four tablespoons of cold-pressed fats, like olive oil. The rest of the pyramid included five to nine servings of vegetables a day, five to seven ounces of "protein foods" (which included meat, eggs, nuts and beans), and two to three servings of dairy. Sugar should be kept to no more than ten percent of your caloric intake, and white flour was lumped into the "junk food," which was to be consumed rarely or never.[31]

The organization that hired her was the U.S. Department of Agriculture (USDA). Unfortunately, USDA's job is to support our farmers, not provide us with sound nutritional advice.

So for reasons that had absolutely nothing to do with health, we were told to eat bread, pasta, and cereal to our heart's content, and get rid of eggs, butter, and whole milk.

All of which is to say that, an entire nation changed its way of eating based on a combination of scant evidence and political economics.

If you were like me, you followed the recommendations, buying fat-free yogurt, drinking skim milk, eating cereals and bread (whole grain if you were trying to stay healthy). And you consumed what we now know was about five to ten times the number of carbs your body can really handle. As one researcher said, "Our diet is mismatched with our biochemistry."[32]

At some point, your physiology just became overloaded, and you suffered the consequences.

When Food Became Cheap and Addictive

While all this was going on, the big food companies were very busy figuring out how to become more successful (i.e. more profitable). Saving a few pennies per product would increase their profits by hundreds of thousands of dollars or more, so they hired chemists and invested millions in research and development. And it worked like a charm. They substituted inexpensive chemicals that *tasted* like food for ones that had to be (expensively) grown and raised. They increased sugar and salt, because this "food" would be completely unpalatable otherwise. Because both of those compounds are chemical wonders, acting as preservatives to lengthen shelf life, improve consistency, bind ingredients together, etc. They also stimulate the dopamine receptors in your brain, making these processed foods as addictive as heroin or cocaine.

Supermarkets, vending machines, and corner gas stations quickly filled their shelves with "hyper-palatable" items that never go bad and keep you coming back for more. Fast food exploded because it was now easy to keep these food substitutes on hand almost indefinitely and heat them up quickly. Super-sizing and free refills were born. Then came the 99-cent menu to get people in the door. And before we knew it, we were surrounded by food that wasn't actually *food*.

And then they marketed all this to a population that wanted to be modern, and hip, and all the things the commercials told us we would be. Now that women were in the workplace, they told us that we just didn't have any time to cook anymore; and once home economics was taken out of the schools, we didn't know how to anyway. What a joy those instant mixes became, cutting the prep time for brownies down from thirty minutes to five!

And because these foods were formulated to be addictive, we kept coming back for more. We bought the frozen pizza that (like three-quarters of the frozen pizzas on the market today) didn't even use real cheese. We ate low-fat frozen dinners that contained chemicals we didn't recognize, and drank our sodas, filled with the hidden sodium that makes us thirsty to drink more. The serving sizes got larger and larger, and still we'd clean our plates . . . and then we'd order dessert.

When We Took A Seat

The current expression for pointing out the dangers of a sedentary lifestyle is, "Sitting Is The New Smoking."

To everything I've listed above, add in a lifestyle that has many of us driving everywhere and sitting in front of our computers for hours at a time. We all know that exercise burns calories (and that's still true—not everything you learned was wrong), but there's more to it than that. I'll talk more about the physiology of this later in the book, but for now let's just say this: exercise burns glucose. And when you fill your bloodstream with glucose without burning it off, you leave all that glucose (and insulin) sitting there to do its damage.

And now all of this political and commercial control of our diet has come together to create the perfect storm that is this diabetes epidemic.

Calories In, Calories Out

We are all familiar with calories, and there is some truth that eating too many calories causes weight gain. The thing is, you are not a furnace. Let me explain.

The old model of dealing with weight looked at counting calories. A gram of carbohydrates is 4 calories; a gram of fat is 9 calories. So in a calorie-counting world, it would seem logical to eat low fat. The problem is, calories from different foods behave differently in the body.

Even though a gram of carbs is only 4 calories, you have to consider that it also comes with insulin. And the second you put insulin in your bloodstream, you cannot burn fat. A gram of fat, though, doesn't need insulin to metabolize. It breaks down into fuel for your body without triggering insulin, which allows you to burn your fat stores. In fact, in research studies, they show that eating the same amount of calories between low-fat and low-carb diets (meaning, eating higher fat), that those who ate more fat had better weight loss, better cardiovascular markers, and were more satiated and satisfied with their food.[33]

A 2012 study compared groups eating the same amount of calories but in different ratios—one was a high-glycemic diet at 60% carbohydrates, one was a medium-glycemic load at 40%, and one was low-carb, with 60% of the calories coming from fat.[34] The result? The low-carb people burned 300 more calories per day than the others, even though they were all eating the same amount. Sounds crazy, right?

In fact, eating low fat for long periods of time can permanently damage your metabolism. Another study from 2016 followed the contestants of the reality TV show "The Biggest Loser" in 2008.[35] It turns out that such caloric, low-fat restriction while they were on the show had changed their metabolism so significantly that 6 years later, their metabolisms hadn't recovered.

So yes, calories count, but don't be paranoid about fat.

It's Not Really Your Genetics

We inherited two things from our parents: their genes, and their way of life. It takes thousands of years to change genes (they estimate about 10,000 years, actually). But this diabetes epidemic has just shown up in the last 30 years. We don't have a diabetic gene that's just appeared. What you might have is a combination of genes that have existed in your family for many, many generations, but it is only with the exposure to this excess of food that these "genetics" appeared. In fact, in the field of genetics, it's estimated that genetics plays only a 20-30% part in the development of diabetes.

It's far from guaranteed that you'll get diabetes if your mother or father has it, and Type 2 diabetes has proven to be reversible with the right diet changes.

No, this is a man-made crisis. Which is good news, because it means you can "unmake" it.

NUTRITIONAL DEFICIENCIES AND DIABETES

One of the impacts of having Type 2 diabetes is not just that the overload of calories and sugar over time have damaged certain organs and made you insulin resistant, but also that you've used your nutrients while trying to handle all that overload. Over time, you start to deplete whatever stores you had, and since most of us aren't eating great, we start to go into deficiency. More on that in a second . . .

Nutrients involved in the metabolism of all those carbs, as well as making those insulin receptor sites work, include multiple B vitamins, Coenzyme Q10 (CoQ10), magnesium, zinc, chromium, vanadium . . . the list goes on.

So why is that a big deal?

The reason this is significant is because they're starting to see in research that, it's not just the fact that big deficiencies cause problems (think scurvy from not having enough Vitamin C), but also that long-term, low-level deficiencies contribute to the degenerative diseases we're seeing. In multiple animal studies, they saw that these subclinical deficiencies caused osteoporosis, dementia, and cancer,[36,37,38] and it could be argued that we're already seeing this play out in humans.

One study noted that, "the prevalence of nutrient deficiency is higher in overweight, obese, and morbidly obese compared to normal weight patients, suggesting that obese patients may consume an excess of dietary energy, but they may not meet their entire essential nutrient needs."[39] And I wouldn't say that it's just people with weight issues—this is happening in with nearly all of my patients. Magnesium, selenium, iron, chromium, and zinc were all highlighted in this study, and considering that magnesium is involved in over 300 enzyme reactions, and zinc is implicated in at least 200, imagine how much is NOT happening in your body when you have even mild deficiencies.

It's not accurate to say that only carb intake or diabetes causes this, though. Anything that causes us to not have enough nutrients contributes to this problem—such as eating a lot of processed foods that are "empty" in nutrients, not eating whole or real foods, drinking a lot of alcohol, eating conventionally raised (non-organic) fruits and vegetables (the soil these days is too poor for the produce to have much nutrition, so buy organic when you can). But also, eating low fat foods (there are vitamins in fat, and they help you absorb minerals), eating only muscle meat, and not eating organ meats (like liver) or making soup out of the bones like traditional cultures... the list goes on and on. You even get nutrient deficiencies with taking some medications. It's well known, for example, that metformin causes B12 deficiency![40,41]

So every time you choose to eat a real food instead of a processed one, or you pass on the dessert, or you eat dinner at home (a real dinner, not a microwave one!) you are not only stopping this loss of nutrients but also adding them back in.

UNDERSTANDING PROPER NUTRITION

Macronutrient Breakdowns

Macronutrient is just a fancy term for the kind of nutrient that provides calories. There are three kinds: protein, fat, and carbohydrates.

Protein

Proteins are primarily broken down in the stomach and require proper levels of stomach acid to do so. You find protein in animal products (meat, eggs, and dairy), soy, nuts, seeds, and beans.

I'm not going to spend a lot of time on this one, because protein doesn't have a huge impact on blood sugar—unless you eat a lot of it. The one thing I will say: soy is actually very difficult to digest and can cause all sorts of problems, ranging from digestive distress, to hypothyroidism, and to preventing absorption of nutrients. This includes tofu, soymilk, soy cheeses, soy yogurts, and soy "meats." The exception is soy that's been *fermented* because the fermentation process neutralizes the harmful compounds. This means that miso, tempeh, and soy sauce are much easier to digest.

Fats

Fats are found in animal products, plant oils, and many are added to processed foods. There are four main types:

- **Saturated:** solid at room temperature and very resistant to going rancid. These are the fats often associated with meat, dairy, and eggs, though coconut oil and nuts have quite a bit, too.

- **Monounsaturated:** liquid at room temperature and vulnerable to becoming rancid. Olive oil is a top provider of monounsaturated fat.

- **Polyunsaturated:** found in very small quantities and extremely vulnerable to becoming rancid. Commonly found in nut, flaxseed, and fish oils.

- **Trans Fats/Hydrogenated Fats:** these are extremely *dangerous* and absolutely contribute to heart disease, which is why they are being removed from the food industry. Found in anything with the word "hydrogenated" on the label, such as refrigerated dough (stuff that comes in a tube: crescent rolls and frozen cookie dough), chips, supermarket cakes, and icing—basically any place butter would have been used in the past. They are very difficult for the body to clear. It takes about 90 days to clear this kind of fat, so *avoid it at all costs.*

By the way, none of the foods that exist in nature have purely one type of fat in them. They will always have a mix of both saturated and unsaturated. For example, beef fat actually has as much unsaturated fat in it as you'd find in olive oil.

A few decades back, we got paranoid about saturated fats, because researchers thought that saturated fat raised LDL, and they saw that people with heart disease had high LDL. From that, they concluded that saturated fat must cause heart disease.

The thing is, they never really tested their theory. They never looked for people with high LDL who don't have heart disease, which it turns out is quite common. If they had not muddled things up like this, they might have looked for the other things consumed by people with heart disease that might have been the real culprit.

It turns out that not all LDL is bad. There's a light, fluffy "good" kind (type A), which is the precursor to your hormones. (Drive your cholesterol down too far and you can't make testosterone, for example!) And there's a small, dense "bad" kind, which makes plaque. And what contributes to the small, dense bad kind? You guessed it—sugar, white flour, and processed seed oils like corn oil, soy oil, cottonseed oil, etc. Eat more of those things, and you drive up your total cholesterol, regardless of your fat (or type of fat) intake.

Fortunately, the medical community is starting to wise up to this fact. For a while now, there's been general agreement that hydrogenated fats and trans-fatty acids are bad news, and in recent years they've started to consider the possibility that saturated fat might not be. And gradually, the focus on LDL is shifting towards triglycerides, which is a much better measure of an individual's risk of cardiovascular disease.

For more information on this, check out Gary Taubes' feature in *The New York Times,* "What If It's All Been A Big, Fat Lie?"[42] or Time magazine's 2014 cover story, "Ending the War on Fat."[43]

With all that in mind, let's take a look at some of the healthy fats out there:

- Fats in meat or dairy (including red meat and butter)
- Chicken skin
- Coconut oil
- Nuts and seeds
- Eggs
- Avocado
- Seed oils (olive, peanut, sesame, etc.)
- Lard

Lard? How is that a healthy fat? This one always shocks people a bit, as we've fallen hook, line and sinker, for the "lard clogs your pipes" way of thinking. But lard is actually in the same category as olive oil, primarily a monounsaturated fat, and it's come back as a good cooking oil. ("Lard: The New Health Food" in *Food and Wine* magazine is a fantastic introduction to straightening out our misunderstandings about lard.)[44]

Coconut oil is particularly helpful when you're changing your diet in the way we recommend. It's what's known as a "medium-chain fatty acid," which means that your body won't store it as fat, but uses it just like a carbohydrate— meaning it's quick energy! We like to promote the use of this oil whenever you're cooking your food, but we've had people who stir it into their coffee and tea for a quick pick-me-up, or even lick it off a spoon! The refined kind doesn't taste like coconut like the unrefined does, but they both work the same, and there's no weird chemistry in the refining process- it only means they removed the coconut proteins. So pick whichever tastes better to you.

Fats to be avoided:

- Partially hydrogenated vegetable fats (trans-fats)
- Unsaturated oils that are not cold pressed or expeller pressed

Commercially prepared seed oils (corn, canola, vegetable, etc.) found in grocery stores are *NOT safe to eat.* They use high temperatures and chemical solvents to economically extract the oils, and in the process they become damaged and rancid. The offensive smells are removed prior to bottling, but the free radicals are still present. These oils are one of the leading causes of heart disease.

Carbohydrates

And finally, we have reached the real culprit of diabetes: carbohydrates.

Carbohydrates are quick forms of energy for the body to use. They convert easily to glucose, the main fuel of the body, of which 30% is used for brain function. This is why you have difficulty concentrating, or you get tired or irritable when your blood sugar is low—because your brain is literally starving.

One thing to note is that your body doesn't actually need carbohydrates to get all its nutrients. Carbs are quick and easy to use as fuel, but your body can obtain all of its energy and nutrients from protein and fats. This is vital to remember, because the general recommendation about how you should always have a carb on your plate has contributed to the mess we're in.

There are two kinds of carbs: simple/refined (also known as simple sugars) and complex/unrefined. Simple carbs are anything that ends with an "-ose" (sucrose—which is white sugar—glucose, fructose, lactose, dextrose, etc.) as well as white, refined flour. Most of these simple sugars cause your blood sugar to rise rapidly and increase insulin levels as a reaction.

Complex carbs are basically chains of glucose bound together, and are found in whole grains and starches—e.g., potatoes, pasta, and rice. They're bound together with fiber and other nutrients, which help to slow down absorption and feed your body in other ways. However, they still cause blood sugar and insulin levels to rise.

People often forget that vegetables are carbs as well, albeit low-count carbs! And, of course, they also have fiber. I had a patient email me once, saying that if they weren't going to eat grains, where would they get their fiber? I answered, "From the increased amount of vegetables you'll be eating!"

In fact, one of the things I tell my patients is that we waste valuable stomach space on bread, when we should be eating more vegetables.

We've often been told that if it's a "good carb" that it's okay to eat it, or that if it's "whole grain" or "low glycemic" that it's fine. But one thing I tell my patients is that once your system is "broken," the general rules no longer apply. For someone who is insulin-resistant or diabetic, these carbs can still cause an overreaction of insulin, which is why using the glycemic index is not recommended by the American Diabetes Association. Additionally, we have no idea about serving sizes—just because brown rice is a lower glycemic food doesn't mean that eating a cup of it is healthy!

So just remember that all vegetables have carbs too, but the green ones and the non-starchy colorful ones (e.g., broccoli, carrots, and beets) don't have much. No one ever got diabetes from eating too many carrots!

SUGAR: WHAT'S IN A NAME?

Fructose

Before we go on, we need to talk about a special sugar: fructose.

There's a lot of confusion regarding fructose, because it seems like it must be okay. It's found naturally in fruit, right?

Well, yes and no. Fruit would have been fine if we'd left it the way we found it. But we didn't. We took that orange and stuck it in a juicer along with several other oranges and made orange juice, thinking that it was just as healthy. But it's not. Because when you do that, you're getting all of the sugar and none of the healthy fiber.

In the concentrations found in juice, or high-fructose corn syrup, the fructose goes directly to your liver and metabolizes in the same pathways as alcohol. Some of you might have also heard of fatty liver disease, and some of you may even have received this diagnosis. In the past, it was mostly associated with a high intake of alcohol, which damaged the liver, causing fatty liver disease, which led to cirrhosis of the liver. But that's not what's happening these days. That's right—drink too much alcohol and you get fatty liver disease; eat or drink too much fructose and you get non-alcoholic fatty liver disease (NAFLD).[45] This can ultimately lead to cirrhosis and liver cancer, and like I mentioned earlier, is far more prevalent than people realize. It is thought that up to 75% of obese people have NAFLD,[46] with 8 out of 10 of these people showing normal liver enzymes on a blood test, making this condition extremely difficult to detect.

So while glucose and insulin are hugely damaging in large amounts, fructose is just as bad, albeit in a different way. Altogether, the physiological impact is pretty astounding. Fructose increases your triglycerides and increases your visceral fat (which has been linked to insulin resistance and heart disease).[47,48] It makes you hungrier, which makes you eat more.[49] It causes your body to make the small, dense LDL particles that cause plaques.[50] And it drives NAFLD, which can ultimately lead to cirrhosis and liver cancer.

Your body will release insulin because it thinks carbohydrates are on the way, even if they're not!

Turns out that it's also the high caloric intake and fructose that causes this issue, and it's now being seen as not limited just to the liver. There's also fatty pancreas,[51,52] fatty heart,[53,54] and even fatty tongue! Oh, and this fat isn't the visceral fat that you might have heard of, that is AROUND the organs—this fat is actually fat droplets IN the cells of the organs. Basically, when faced with this overload of calories, your body desperately puts all the excess, not just into fat cells, but into organ cells as well. Since the organs aren't designed for that overload, organ function starts to break down.

It's now being recognized how prevalent this is: 70-85% of Type 2 diabetics have NAFLD.[55] And it's not just limited to people with weight issues or diabetes—it's been shown that fatty liver/organ disease has its highest prevalence in people with poor insulin sensitivity.[56]

Different Types of Sweeteners

"But I don't drink fruit juice or soda!", my patients will say. That's great, except those aren't the only places where fructose is found in high concentrations. People are always trying to find some substitute for sugar—some miracle sweetener that doesn't have calories or cause serious health problems. Let's just say that researchers are still looking for this miracle.

One of the problems with sweeteners is that your body still recognizes the sweet taste no matter what kind of sweetener you might be using. Usually, your body will release insulin because it *thinks* carbohydrates are on the way, even if they're not.

Another problem is that, after years of eating sweet things, the receptors on your tongue are exhausted, and it takes more and more of the sweet flavor to actually taste the sweetness. It takes about two weeks for your tongue to recover. (When it does, your experience of all foods will improve!)

There are at least 61 different names for sugar:

1. Agave nectar
2. Barbados sugar
3. Barley malt
4. Barley malt syrup
5. Beet sugar
6. Brown sugar
7. Buttered syrup
8. Cane juice
9. Cane juice crystals
10. Cane sugar
11. Caramel
12. Carob syrup
13. Castor sugar
14. Coconut palm sugar
15. Coconut sugar
16. Confectioner's sugar
17. Corn sweetener
18. Corn syrup
19. Corn syrup solids
20. Date sugar
21. Dehydrated cane juice
22. Demerara sugar
23. Dextrin
24. Dextrose
25. Evaporated cane juice
26. Free-flowing brown sugars
27. Fructose
28. Fruit juice
29. Fruit juice concentrate
30. Glucose
31. Glucose solids
32. Golden sugar
33. Golden syrup
34. Grape sugar
35. HFCS (High-Fructose Corn Syrup)
36. Honey
37. Icing sugar
38. Invert sugar
39. Malt syrup
40. Maltodextrin
41. Maltol
42. Maltose
43. Mannose
44. Maple syrup
45. Molasses
46. Muscovado
47. Palm sugar
48. Panocha
49. Powdered sugar
50. Raw sugar
51. Refiner's syrup
52. Rice syrup
53. Saccharose
54. Sorghum Syrup
55. Sucrose
56. Sugar (granulated)
57. Sweet Sorghum
58. Syrup
59. Treacle
60. Turbinado sugar
61. Yellow sugar

Pretty much every "sugar" on here is some combination of glucose and fructose. And as we've seen, glucose causes that insulin reaction that leads to insulin resistance and prevents you from losing weight, while fructose damages the liver like alcohol.

So let's take a look at some of these:

Regular table sugar, whether it's white or brown or raw or organic, is a 50-50 mix of fructose and glucose. (Sucrose is just a fructose and glucose molecule stuck together.) So if you eat a diet that has any sugar in it at all, you're getting fructose in that. And while people often demonize high-fructose corn syrup (HFCS) and think "real organic cane sugar" is a better alternative, the two actually aren't very biochemically different. That "real organic cane sugar" is a 50-50 mix of fructose and glucose, compared to HFCS, which is around 55-45.

Honey is basically the same, too. With honey you are getting a few extra compounds that offer some nutrients, but most of it is still just a mixture of glucose and fructose. Like I tell my patients, we used to have to fight bees for their honey, so that naturally limited our intake of it. Now we just pull it out of our cupboards. So while it's better than most of the stuff on this list, it's still something to limit.

Agave nectar is marketed as being a healthy alternative, but it is anything but. The agave root has a starch called inulin (not to be confused with insulin), which is only about 10% as sweet as sugar. Because it's not sweet enough by itself, the naturally occurring sweetener in it (fructose) has to be concentrated into a syrup that has about 90% fructose, which we're told is healthy because it's "low glycemic." Except the glycemic index only tells you how quickly something dumps glucose into your bloodstream. Since it's only got 10% glucose it definitely qualifies, but that doesn't mean it's good for you. Just like juicing an orange, you've removed all the fiber and are pounding back the fructose.

There are some other seemingly healthy sweetener options that are actually anything but healthy. **Coconut sugar** is 38-48% fructose depending on the brand, which is almost the same as regular sugar, gram-for-gram; and **crystalline fructose,** as you may have guessed by the name, is 98% fructose, 2% glucose.

Then there are all the non-sugar sweeteners, most of which should be *avoided like the plague.* Take **aspartame,** for instance. Out of all food additives passed by the FDA, aspartame took the longest. It's been shown in studies to cause brain lesions, among other nasty issues. I've helped countless patients who have cleared up chronic and severe health problems just by cutting out aspartame, so avoid this one at all costs. **Sucralose** (often the kind in the little yellow packets) is a sucrose molecule with chlorine added to it. Yum.

Let's be honest, though. The problem with cutting out sugar is that we still want it, right? Don't worry, there are many good alternatives, and you might not even notice the difference.

Stevia is one sweetener that is okay—it's from a plant and is about 300% the sweetness of sugar, so a little goes a long way. Although, keep in mind that it is still relatively new, so there is less safety information on it. However, it's been used in Japan for over 30 years, and so far, it appears to be safe from any toxic side effects. It's one of two sweeteners that doesn't cause an increase in insulin, so if you have to use a sweetener, this might be the one. Truvia™ and Pure Via™ are commercial forms that have been processed to remove the slight aftertaste.

Xylitol is another sweetener that can work. It's got about half the calories of sugar, has the same sweetness, and like stevia doesn't cause an insulin reaction. It can be used just like sugar, cooks the same, doesn't have any weird aftertastes, is actually good for your teeth, and is easily bought in the store. The one downside is that it can have a laxative effect if used in large quantities. Don't freak out about this too much—you've probably already had it in sugar-free mints or chewing gum. As long as you don't overdo it, this is a great sweetener to use, and it's my go-to for baking things like pumpkin pie or when I feel like adding a little sweetness to my tea.

Monk Fruit, also known as Luo Han Guo or Lohan fruit, has been used for centuries in China as a sweetener but also is known as the "longevity fruit" for its anti-aging properties, as a cough remedy, for constipation, and as a diabetes treatment. Wow!

The compounds in monk fruit are what give it all these benefits, and when those compounds are concentrated, you get all the benefits without having to eat the fruit with its carb count. You're probably going to start seeing more and more monk fruit based sweeteners in the future, as it's safe for diabetics, and a lot of companies are looking for good alternatives to the chemical artificial sweeteners.

Always keep in mind, though: the less you trigger the sweet taste for yourself, the faster your body begins to reset itself, and the faster you get healthy!

PART 2 — HOW TO PREVENT OR REVERSE TYPE 2 DIABETES

STEP 1: GET YOUR PANTRY READY

To prepare for eating healthier, we first want you to get familiar with what's already in your kitchen. Open your refrigerator and cabinets and take a look, and answer the following questions:

- Are there a lot of boxes, bags, and cans of food?

- What's in them?

- What kind of cooking oils and seasonings have you been using?

- What do they have in them?

- When you're hungry, what do you typically reach for?

- If you haven't cooked food at home in a while, how old would you say the stuff is in your pantry and cabinets?

- What's in your freezer, and how old is it?

Now, look at the labels of all the things you eat regularly, and answer these questions:

- How many have the words "diet" or "lite" on them?

- How many have the words "fat free" or "low calorie"?

- How many have the word "hydrogenated" in the ingredients?

- How many of them have ingredients with the words "sugar," "syrup," or anything from that list of 61 different names for sugar?

All these different labels are as confusing as they are plentiful. A lot of them *imply* "healthy" when, in fact, they are not. Remember, a lot of those ingredients are there to make that food more addictive, or to make it last forever on a shelf.

To be clear, it's not necessary to "fuss" with food, or make an entire meal every time you need to eat. You don't need to clean out your cabinets completely. The trick to becoming healthier is to begin incorporating quick, easy, and healthy options into your everyday life.

But you should be looking at the labels when you go to the grocery store, and be wary of the "tricks of the food trade" so you can stay away from the hidden hazards.

With that in mind, here are some of the staples that are good to have on hand and some others that you want to stay away from. When you go shopping, it's vital that you don't automatically buy the high-carb foods and snacks that you have in the past. KEEP THOSE THINGS OUT OF YOUR HOUSE, and you'll notice it's a lot easier to make good choices.

Things to Get Rid of (or Never Buy Again)

- Vegetable oil, corn oil, soy oil, canola oil
- Fruit juices
- Instant mixes with more than one or two ingredients (think of those "meals-in-a-box" that you just add

meat or chicken, as well as those packages of pasta or rice that became an instant, "just-add-water" side dish—those are what types of things we're after here, as opposed to powdered milk or oats)

- Candy, cookies, and chips
- Anything with "hydrogenated" in the list of ingredients
- Packaged snacks that use refined or bleached flour
- Soft drinks
- Frozen/TV dinners: In general, you'll want to avoid items with a long list of ingredients that you can't easily identify, and if what you're eating has any kind of added sugar or sweetener in it, try to find a version without it.

Things to Stock Up On

Cold- or expeller-pressed olive oil, coconut oil (refined or unrefined), sesame oil, peanut oil, and avocado oil are all good cooking oils.

Carbonated water is fine, and helps satisfy (or reduce) the soft-drink habit for a lot of people. They come in many flavors now, so pick a couple you like.

Shirataki noodles (also known as "miracle noodles") are a great alternative to pasta. They are made from a Japanese yam that has no calories, no carbs, no gluten, and no fat. They are simply fiber. You can buy them in your local Asian grocery, or online (miraclenoodle.com or asianfoodgrocer. com). You can find them in different shapes—from round noodles to flat noodles to "rice."

Nuts make a great snack. Nut butters are also great. Justin's® Nut Butters come in to-go packs, so you can keep them in a purse, backpack, or gym bag, but jars of almond or peanut butter are great for home. Again, look at the ingredients, though. Most of the famous brands (and even the "natural" varieties of them) have sugar and/or one of the oils that are in our no-no list.

Water, green tea, white tea, and black tea are all really healthy to drink, and if you like red wine, have some (just in moderation!).

Again, the whole point of this is that it works within your current lifestyle, because if it doesn't, you're not going to want to make it work. So make the items that work for you part of your stash, and if you find yourself struggling, continue to look for something that works.

STEP 2: THE 7-DAY BLOOD SUGAR REBOOT

There are three main parts to the 7-Day Challenge:

1) Eat 60 grams of carbs per day, excluding green and other non-starchy vegetables.
2) Eat every 3 hours.
3) Include fat with everything you eat, no exception.

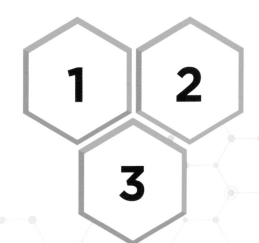

This is not meant to be a "no-carb" diet—this is meant to work in real life, like eating out or eating with friends. And I didn't pick 60 grams arbitrarily—a researcher in Germany, named Wolfgang Lutz, saw that if you didn't want to end up diabetic at the end of your life, you would want to average about 72 grams per day,[57] with maybe a bit more if you were active all the time. Since most people at this point have run out of points, 72 grams is still too much, and we've found 60 grams seems to work better.

Carb Counting Made Easy

Here's the list of items whose carbs you need to count:

Grain-based Foods, such as:	
• Bread	• Breakfast bars/granola bars/energy bars
• Crackers/Chips	
• Cereal/Granola	• Oatmeal
• Bran	• Pasta
	• Rice
Desserts, including:	
• Candy	• Pastries
• Baked goods	• Cookies/cakes
Drinks like:	
• Fruit juices	• Soda
• Milk	• Alcoholic beverages
The Following Grocery Items:	
• Fruit	• Corn (including popcorn)
• Beans	
• Potatoes (*ALL* varieties)	

And of course, anything with a label including sugar, or any of its many euphemisms, including (but not limited to) honey, corn syrup, high fructose corn syrup, agave nectar, evaporated cane syrup, etc. (Remember that list we gave you earlier!)

Notice that this is a list of carb-dense foods, not "bad" foods. That's why it includes things like beans, which have some protein but also have carbs, and healthier foods like oatmeal and sweet potatoes, which have tons of nutrients and fiber but are still carb-dense.

Also, you may have heard that tomatoes, cucumbers, and avocados are technically fruits. While that's true (the official definition of a fruit is the flesh that surrounds a seed) those aren't the fruits we're talking about here. Yes, they have carbs in them, but as with carrots, nobody got diabetes from eating too many avocados. What we're talking about are the things you traditionally think of when you think of a fruit: i.e., the sweet ones. If it's something that people might cover in chocolate or whipped cream and serve for dessert, then that's a fruit. So eat as many tomatoes and cucumbers as you want.

Net Carbs: Much Ado about Nothing

There's all this confusion of "net carbs" versus regular carbs. Net carbs sound great—take a food labeled with net carbs and it takes the "regular" carb load down significantly. Free carbs! Sounds too good to be true!

And it is. The definition of net carbs is simply the grams of total carbohydrates in a portion of food minus its grams of fiber. Now, fiber is great for a variety of reasons, and one of these is that fiber slows the absorption of glucose. This means you don't get a glucose spike, but this does NOT mean that this food doesn't have carbs. When the label says it has 25 grams of carbs, but only 5 grams of net carbs, this doesn't mean it magically lost 20 grams of carbs. It's basically just saying that the fiber is slowing down the absorption. But the issue is still that there's glucose in the system causing an insulin reaction. Insulin is released REGARDLESS, and that's the whole issue, or what we're trying to avoid.

Net carbs looks like magic math, doesn't it? Don't fall for it— deal with the *total number* of grams of carbs only.

 ## 60 Grams a Day—In Action

You're going to look at two things—is this food on the list above? And how much are you having? If it's not on the list, then it doesn't need to be counted. **Count only what's on the list.**

So how fast does 60g go? Well, a piece of bread is about 20g of carbs. A banana is 29. A serving of rice is typically about 1 cup and it's 45 g. A glass of orange juice (8 oz.) is 26. Do you see how quickly this adds up if you're not paying attention?

If it came in a package, then it should be easy for you to determine how many grams of carbohydrates you're having. For the produce, you may have to look it up. Here are a couple of good online calculators that will include name brands, if that's helpful: www.myfitnesspal.com and www.loseit.com.

Let's look at this in action. Say you have some oatmeal for breakfast—the serving size of old-fashioned, cook-it-yourself oatmeal is ½ cup dry, and it has 27 grams of carbs. So did you eat just a half-cup? Or did you have more? Did you put raisins in it? Or sprinkle some sugar on it? How about some milk? All these have carbs in them. Add all of this together, and the number might be a bit shocking.

But what if you had scrambled eggs? That's pure protein, and also not on the list. You sprinkled a little cheddar cheese on it, but cheese is not milk, has very little lactose (depending on the type), and minimal carbs, if any, which is why cheese is not on the list. You added half an avocado (also not on the list), a little tomato, and put it on a bed of spinach (none of which are on the list). Nothing in this breakfast impacted your 60-gram allotment of the day. Great! Not to mention delicious!

Let me repeat: the only thing you're counting here is your grams of carbs. Not fat intake, not calories, nor protein intake. Just grams of carbs.

Literally, if it's not on that list, don't count it.

And remember—this doesn't include green vegetables, so eat as much of them as you want.

ADA Recommendations: Where's the Logic?

It seems quite clear, right? Carbohydrates turn into sugar in your blood, and if you want to drop the sugar in your blood, you should eat fewer carbohydrates. This is so logical that back before insulin was discovered, (they didn't see it in the blood yet, but they could test for it in urine), this was how doctors treated high blood sugar—with a diet that was 70% fat, 8% carbohydrate. That's right—a mostly fat diet brought these Type 1 diabetics back into normal ranges.[58]

Which makes it hard to understand, then, why the American Diabetes Association's recommendations are 45-60 grams of carbs *per meal.* No wonder the average person can't get their blood sugar handled or their diabetes reversed!

2 | 3-Hour Intermissions

When your system is primed for sugar and carbs, the moment your blood sugar drops and you get hungry, your brain starts looking for carbs to feed it. Those are the times you crave sugar. People always think that they just don't have willpower, but that's not it—it's just that you're hungry! And so, until your blood sugar learns to stabilize itself, you need to help your body along, and avoid getting into that low-blood sugar state. That means eating something every 2-3 hours, or before you get hungry. This is vital.

If you find that every three hours isn't enough, and you're still getting those cravings or you're still getting irritable or tired before you eat, then increase the frequency. We had a patient once who monitored herself closely and discovered that the 2½-hour mark is when she started getting tired and cranky. When she ate every 2 hours, she felt great. So that's what she did. Three or four weeks later, she tested herself again, and noticed she could now go 3½ hours before those symptoms kicked in. That's how quickly this can turn around.

Eating something every 2-3 hours, or before you get hungry is VITAL.

As you get healthier, you may see that you can go longer without eating, which is fine as long as you don't get hungry, and then make bad food choices!

In a perfect world, I'd love for people to have relaxed, sit-down meals three times a day and to not have to eat in this grazing mode that so many of us do. As you get healthier, consider trying to move more towards real meals, and move away from too much snacking and grazing.

Join the Fat Revival

After decades, or a lifetime, of eating low fat, you might struggle with this initially. I know I did. One problem is, we don't even realize we're doing it anymore. The most popular cut of meat is a boneless, skinless chicken breast. The default milk for your favorite latté is 2%. It's actually quite difficult to find full-fat yogurt because everything on the shelves is typically fat-free or low fat.

But remember that this all started because we took fat out of our diet. So let's put it back in. Eating carrot sticks is okay, but eating carrot sticks with hummus (which has olive oil), or eating a half an apple with almond butter works a whole lot better.

Fat and Carbs: Proportional Harmony

Because fat fills us up. It stabilizes our blood sugar. It gives us consistent energy over time, keeping our brain fed and our willpower strong. It also provides vital nutrients we need to restore our blood vessels and our cell membranes, so it allows us to access the nutrients in the food we're eating. And it adds back in the flavor we've been craving after all this low-fat stuff.

Now, you get to have all of that wonderful, real food back again. No more skim milk in your coffee—use half-and-half. Skip the turkey bacon and get the real stuff. Throw away that almost-like-real-butter spread. Eat eggs! Put butter on those steamed vegetables, and add some cheese to your salad. Welcome back to the world of real food.

Sometimes people think I'm recommending that they eat more meat, which is not what I'm saying. I said before, there are only three nutrients that provide calories—carbohydrates, proteins, and fats—and we've spent decades taking fat out. Now I'm telling you to take a lot of the carbohydrates out instead, and add the fat back in. Yes, you can also add in protein, but we're focusing on the fats—nuts, olive oil, beans, avocado, dairy, coconut, all of those have fat in them, and they're all incredibly nutritious.

I always hope that people will increase their vegetable intake, because no one in our society eats enough vegetables. So add those in too. As long as you're using fat instead of carbohydrates to fill yourself up, you'll start feeling much better soon.

Here's the thing, though—you don't get to add in fat and NOT eat less carbs. Research is correct when it says that a high fat diet is unhealthy *but this is when someone has high blood sugar.* You cannot simply add fat into the diet and not also reduce the carbs.

So again, the three parts of this are:

1) Eat 60 grams of carbs per day.

2) Eat about every 3 hours.

3) Eat fat with everything.

01
Eat Fat.
Feel Full.

02
Eat Fat.
Stabilize Your Sugar.
Control Your Cravings.

03
Eat Fat.
Maintain Energy.
Feed Your Brain.
Strengthen Your Willpower.

04
Eat Fat.
Access the Vital
Nutrients in the
Foods You're Eating.

STEP 3: **BEYOND THE 7-DAY REBOOT**

Most diets end up being temporary, and with good reason. Who can put up with eating only cabbages or grapefruit every day? Who wants to count points or drink weight loss shakes forever?

This plan is different. I'm really trying to teach people how to eat for the rest of their lives, because it's not just a matter of getting your blood sugar down to normal; it's to give you some tools to prevent the diseases that are so rampant today. So, here are a couple of things to keep in mind.

First, you won't have to count carbs forever. I certainly don't anymore. But I've been doing this for a while, so I've got a pretty good internal calculator at this point. I know how many of those potatoes I can eat before hitting my limit. Yes, I still check the labels at the grocery store, particularly if it's something I haven't eaten before, but I'm not using a notepad to write it all down.

If I'm going to a birthday party with a homemade cake and real buttercream frosting, then I know I'll probably have some. (If it's a supermarket cake I have no problem resisting—they don't even taste good to me anymore.) But I come to the party not having had many carbs that day, or yesterday, or the whole week, and I'll go right back to eating correctly tomorrow. Once in awhile, an indulgence is okay. It's when we find ourselves having sugar every day, or multiple times a week, or every "special occasion" (how many birthdays happen in your office every month?) that we find ourselves in trouble.

The second thing is, you're not going to be perfect at this after a week. In fact, you're not going to be perfect at this after a month. I say this for two reasons. First, you've been eating a certain way your entire life. If you're forty, that means you've spent 39½ years probably developing this particular habit. You can't expect that to change in a week. Second, we don't live in a culture of health. It's a lot harder to resist temptation when someone's bringing donuts into the break room every day than if they're not.

On a practical level, we find a ton of people who are able to make this change for a week or two, but then they go to a party, or they decide to have dessert, and then before they know it, they're eating exactly the way they did before. This is normal.

Now, some people just stay there, and keep eating that way, using reasons like "I just can't control myself," or "It just tastes so good!" But the only difference between people who succeed at this and people who don't is that the people who succeed get right back on the wagon if they fall off. So what happens if you went to happy hour and had a whole bunch of chips and other foods that don't work? In your next meal, just go back to eating the way we recommend here. That's it.

What this looks like in real life is this: you'll do great the first week or two. Then something will happen, like a dinner party where you had dessert, and then next morning you will then have a choice—have scrambled eggs with cheese on a bed of spinach? Or waffles? By now, you might be making good choices about food half the time. *Just keep practicing.* Soon it will be 60% of the time. Then 70%. And before you know it, you'll be making good choices more than 90% of the time, and you'll have achieved the results you've been looking for!

It's just a matter of practice.

Breaking the Food Addiction

Overcoming food addictions can be tough—that's why they're called "addictions" and it's why there are rat studies showing that sugar feeds the same brain centers as cocaine.[33] The best way to break your food addiction is to take things one step at a time.

One way we do this in our clinic is we have people write a food journal for a week, and without making any modifications, we have them just circle the things that have sugar in them. You might have to read the labels to find out. The second week, we have them fill out the journal again, circle the foods with sugar and carbs, and then look up the carb counts, and total them up each day. This is just to give you the "lay of the land" so you know what you're doing, instead of living in some fantasy world of carb intake.

The BEST way to break your food addiction is to take things ONE step at a time.

Sometimes people would like to avoid this step, but we tell them it's like the movie *The Matrix*—you have to see what's actually going on before you make changes.

This doesn't necessarily mean cutting something out cold turkey, changing things a little at a time, and finding a replacement. For example, let's say you drink six sodas a day. The first step might be to cut it down to five, but ALSO to look at when you drink them. Is it in the morning when you're tired? In the afternoon as a "pick-me-up"? Is it because that's the only thing in the fridge at work? Or it's a "treat" because of a stressful day?

So let's say you cut it down to five sodas a day. You can start replacing some of the soda intake with flavored sparkling water. After a week, try for four sodas a day, and adding in more sparkling water, maybe trying a new flavor. Another week, down to three. See how it goes?

Sometimes we eat those foods because they're all that's around. What you might not know is that these are engineered to cause addiction, so eating or drinking them will make you want more and make it harder to stop. Without just taking them out, is it possible to get some replacements for these snack foods? Absolutely! That's why we have a Snack & Dessert Recipes book to help you with this!

Another thing I tell my patients is that they are not the only ones who have had this issue and that there is someone, somewhere on the internet, who has solved their problem for them. So if you're looking for some work-around for a favorite food, chances are you just have to find your answer on the web.

Eating Your Way Out of a Sticky Situation

You might be wondering if there is anything you can actually DO food-wise if you have started to have some of the more significant issues that can come with diabetes, like neuropathy pain and problems with the eyes and kidneys.

In the old way of thinking, your arteries and veins and capillaries are seen as tubes that transport blood around the body. While that's true, scientists have learned a lot more about what's going on in there than you might realize. It's actually one of the hottest fields in research, because they're realizing that the endothelial lining of the blood vessels controls not just the obvious, like hypertension, but also arteriosclerosis, angiogenesis (the circulation that feeds cancers), inflammation . . . the list is long.[59] Even back in 1997 they suspected that damage to the endothelial lining could be a cause of diabetes![60]

It's damaged by high blood sugar (surprise!), but also age, gender, high cholesterol, high inflammation, and high homocysteine. Because your circulatory system is so widespread, having a damaged endothelial lining can result in damage to ANY PART OF THE BODY WHERE CAPILLARIES

ARE VITAL. These are the places where diabetics have the most trouble, because of the "sticky blood" that occurs with high blood sugar blocks the blood flow as well as damages the endothelial lining—kidneys and eyes are the most well-known, but it's the same mechanism for the circulatory damage that ultimately contributes to amputation.

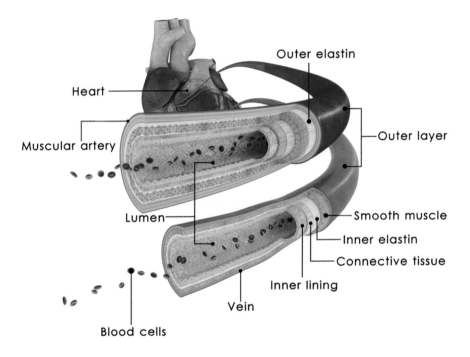

So what can you do? Well, besides actively and aggressively managing your blood sugar, there is some evidence that consistently eating the foods below can help with microcirculation. The trick is, though, that it has to be consistently. Not 2 or 3 times a week, *but every day for several months.*

We had a patient do this for 18 months and saw remarkable changes! We call it the 5-Point Blood Flow Fix, (wow, that's a mouthful, but it works!)

Here are the five foods:

5-Point Blood Flow Fix

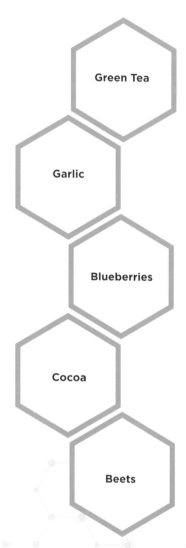

Green tea: You need to drink 3-4 cups per day. This can be cold or hot or flavored, and it doesn't have to be a specific kind.

Garlic: One clove per day. If you absolutely have to, you can use a supplement. If you eat the raw clove, you must either chew it a bit or cut into bits with a knife or make holes with a fork to release the enzymes needed to break it down to its active constituents.

Blueberries or other berries: 2-3 ounces a day. Bilberries would be especially good, although they can be harder to find.

Cocoa: This does not mean milk chocolate. This means either dark chocolate (above 70%) or using cocoa powder that doesn't have sweetener in it. The amount you'll use varies depending on what form you're using.

Beets: At least 2-3 ounces per day as well (we actually just say to have "some every day" in our office!) It's acceptable to use a beet juice concentrate or supplement if you're using one.

Some of you might want stricter guidelines than "some" but it's not so much the exact amount as it is the consistency over time that makes the difference here. This actually holds true for taking nearly any supplement.

Exercise: Fast and Effective

Exercise is far and away, without question, the *fastest* way to reverse diabetes. It lowers blood sugar far more effectively than any medication, and it helps people stave off insulin resistance for years, even decades longer than if they didn't exercise at all.

This has nothing to do with burning calories. It's that exercise makes your system work, even when your system might be "broken," whether with diabetes or anything else. Even if your cells are normally resistant to insulin, exercise forces them to accept glucose—taking it out of the blood stream, where it causes damage, and putting it safely into the cells, where it's used for energy. And this doesn't just happen while you exercise, it occurs for several hours *after* exercise as well.[61]

Now, NOT exercising, for even a short period of time, can cause rather drastic changes in the opposite direction. One research study took young healthy men,[62] and made them stay in bed for 9 days. They could only get up for a total of 15 minutes per day, and spent the rest of the time reading, or on a laptop, or resting in some way. Shockingly, in these *healthy* young men, they caused insulin resistance in just 9 days!

Now, you're probably not lying in bed all day—you're getting up and walking around *some*. But without maintaining a lot more activity, getting your blood sugar under control will be hard-to-impossible. Please don't give up on this part!

But the best thing is: exercise works for people with diabetes exactly the same as for people who don't—it overrides the insulin resistance and FORCES the cell to take glucose. That's great news for diabetics!

And the even better news: it doesn't have to take nearly as much time as you think. Contrary to popular belief, spending an hour on the treadmill or elliptical machine is not very effective. Your body gets used to that level of exercise and gets more efficient, translating to fewer calories and less glucose burned.

Workouts: Get More Results in Less Time

It is far more effective to make your body work for less time with more intensity.

That's right—I said less time. There was a 2014 study in which one group did traditional exercise, like walking on a treadmill at a moderate speed for 30 minutes once a day, and the other group, 30 minutes before a meal, did 6 x 1 minute of intense exercise (walking and/or weights) with a recovery between each minute (they called them exercise "snacks"). The results were striking. Blood sugar levels were lower all day for the "exercise snack" group, as well as 24 hours later— far more so than the traditional exercisers.[63]

Riffing off of that, "The Scientific 7-Minute Workout", featured in *The New York Times,* has been a runaway hit. In this series of exercises (with a downloadable app you can use on your phone or tablet to track it), you do the exercise as intensely as you can for 30 seconds, and rest for 10 seconds. It covers everything from arms to legs to abs, all in 7 minutes.[64]

One study took people who were already fit (they were runners) and had them do 30 seconds of exercise at a 3-out-of-10 intensity, 20 seconds of a 6- or 7-out-of-10 intensity, and then 10 seconds of all-out intensity, and then 2 minutes of gentle strolling to rest.[65] They repeated it a handful of times, and did it only 2-3 times per week. And these already-fit people saw improvements in their blood pressure, their racing times, and their ability to recover. If it worked for them, think about how much improvement YOU'D get!

Another study even showed a benefit from ONE minute of exercise! The overweight and out-of-shape participants did 20 seconds of intense riding on an indoor bicycle, followed by 2 minutes of easy pedaling to recover, and repeated this 3 times. Adding in a 2-minute warm-up, and a 3-minute cool-down gives you 10 minutes, and those 10 minutes made a difference—the participants saw a change in endurance, blood sugar control, and muscle structure.[66] Just with 1-minute total of intensity!

And weight training, FYI, works just the same way.

There's a trick, though—the benefit comes with having those intervals be as hard as you can possibly stand it, with much less benefit coming from a halfway effort. But if you're willing to increase the intensity to shorten your workout, then no longer can we say we don't have time to exercise!

Four Basic Exercises

Here's another version here, which also takes 7-8 minutes per day. This one also uses intensity, and incorporates some weight training, using your own body. There are four basic exercises:

> **Get-Ups:** Lay flat on your back and then get up to a standing position. Trust me—these are simple but effective.

Wall-Push-ups: This is like a push-up, just vertical. Walk up to a wall, stand about 2 feet away with your hands outstretched and palms flat on the wall, bend your elbows, and then straighten.

Air Squats: Mimics the movement you would do if you sat in a chair, but in this case there is no chair. You simply squat down as you would to sit in a chair, and then stand back up. Keep your feet pointing forward, and your back straight.

Air Punches: Air Punches are simply standing with one foot in front of the other and then punching the air in front of you as if you were a boxer punching a bag. Alternate between right and left arms.

The workout looks like this:

Day 1	Warm-up: March in place 4 mins. 10 Get-ups. 10 Air Punches
Day 2	20 min walk; moderate pace
Day 3	Warm-up: March in place 4 mins. 10 Wall Push-ups. 10 Air Squats.
Day 4	20 min walk; moderate pace
Day 5	Warm-up: March in place 4 mins. 10 Wall Push-ups. 10 Air Squats. 10 Air Punches (Repeat as many as possible in 8 mins.)
Day 6	20 min walk; moderate pace
Day 7	Rest Day

How do you ramp up the intensity of the workouts? The trick is to complete the work as fast as possible, and make the exercise as intense as you can while still staying within the range of safety. The very best way to do this is to keep track of the time it takes you to complete the exercises. Each time you perform them, try to beat your old time by a few seconds.

As you improve, you can add more reps or more rounds, or move to the floor for the push-ups, or start to use light hand weights.

Intermittent Fasting

Intermittent fasting (IF) is designed to mimic the feasting-famine times of our forefathers, and this can jumpstart your metabolism if you're healthy enough to do it. Typically, lowering your calories, or going too long without eating, or eating a low-calorie diet slows your metabolism down, but intermittent fasting is just that—"occasional"—and it never lets your system slow down, because it doesn't last long enough for that to happen.

There's a long history of intermittent fasting, ranging from different religions that took a day off per week (or several days once or twice a year), to occasionally going without food as a type of "time-off" to give your body a break from food. The benefits of IF are:

- It's a decrease in caloric intake
- It teaches your body to burn fat, not muscle
- It's an increase in growth hormone
- It's easier to burn fat

- It's easier to do than "dieting"

- It improves insulin sensitivity

- It lowers fasting insulin levels

There's a ton of research on how caloric restriction lengthens lifespan, in everything from fruit flies to chimpanzees,[67,68,69] but it's also extremely helpful for cancer prevention,[70,71] making chemotherapy more effective,[72,73] and has even been shown to make a big difference in impacting the insulin resistance of the brain which results in Alzheimer's disease.[74,75] So consider taking on the challenge of some version of fasting, knowing it's helping you in many, many ways.

With Intermittent Fasting, there is no shortage of variations with which to experiment!

Five Days Off, Two Days On—You eat normally (that means this 60g of carbs per day) for five days and "fast" (fewer than 500 calories for women, 600 for men) for two days per week. (The days don't have to be consecutive.) It's very popular in the UK and easier to do for many people.

Eating Two Meals Per Day—This looks like skipping one meal and just eating two meals (in any arrangement—breakfast, lunch, or dinner) per day.

One Day A Week (or every two weeks, or once a month)— Start at lunch, and don't eat until the next day at lunchtime.

12-hour Fasting—Don't eat after dinner, and make sure that you go to bed at least 3 hours after dinner. Then, the next morning, eat breakfast only if it's been 12 hours since you ate dinner. Otherwise, wait until the 12-hour mark.

For ANY method, always make sure you continue to stay hydrated by drinking healthy drinks, like teas and sparkling water.

There are a couple of caveats to watch out for, though:

If you are currently sick, pregnant, underweight, or struggling with fatigue or stress, then IF is not right for you. Fatigue often means that your adrenals are stressed, and going without food will stress them more. It's better to wait until your fatigue is lessened and your energy is better (meaning, when your blood sugar is better-regulated) before you start doing intermittent fasting.

It's also been shown that intermittent fasting may not work the same for women as men, so if you notice that you feel worse doing this, and you've given it a "good college try", then don't continue. Not everything is for everybody.

STEP 4: SMART SUPPLEMENTATION

I could write a whole other book about nutritional supplements (in fact, I do actually teach doctors about this very topic), but since we're focused on blood sugar here, I'm going to resist the temptation to go down that rabbit hole. Instead, I'll just talk about the supplements that have the most impact blood sugar directly.

Herbs and nutritional supplementation are complicated topics and you should probably talk to a health professional that's trained in these healing agents before digging in too deeply. But if you're dealing with Western doctors, prescribing medications that aren't doing much good, it's beneficial to know that there are healthier, safer, and more effective alternatives, with far fewer side effects.

Banaba Leaf

Leaves of the banaba tree, native to Southern Asia, have been used in traditional herbalism for centuries as a remedy for diabetes. Though the first scientific studies documenting banaba's blood sugar-regulating benefits date back to the 1940s, banaba has only recently become a medicinal plant of interest among naturopathic physicians and the health-conscious public, due to the rising diabetes epidemic.

Banaba offers a combination of benefits that are not available in any diabetes drug currently on the market.[76] In your digestive tract, banaba inhibits the breakdown of sugars and starches.[77] It also encourages your cells to absorb available glucose from your bloodstream in an action similar to the way insulin works.[78] Additionally, banaba lowers blood sugar levels by preventing your body from burning fats and proteins for energy, instead favoring the use of glucose.[79] And while insulin promotes fat production, banaba is fat inhibiting,[80] making this powerful plant a useful tool for managing your blood sugar and preventing weight gain.

One of banaba's main active compounds, corosolic acid, takes effect rapidly, lowering blood sugar levels within an hour after you consume it. This is particularly helpful for preventing dangerous post-meal blood sugar surges.[81] In one study, when diabetic and pre-diabetic patients took 10 mg of corosolic acid, their 2-hour post-meal blood sugar levels decreased by 10%.[82] Participants also reported increased energy levels and decreased thirst and hunger. Banaba extract has also been shown to lower fasting blood sugar levels by as much as 30% in Type 2 diabetics within two weeks with daily supplementation.[83] Long-term use of banaba has been shown to improve glucose tolerance and reduce glycation.[84] In one preliminary study, banaba proved as effective as the widely used diabetes drug metformin at reducing elevated blood sugar levels. Banaba has been found to be safe for both short-term and long-term use, with few to no reported adverse effects.[85]

Chromium and Vanadium

Chromium and vanadium are both essential minerals required in trace amounts.

Chromium helps regulate your blood sugar by assisting the function of insulin. It decreases insulin resistance by increasing the number of glucose transport molecules on the surfaces of cells, making them capable of absorbing more glucose.[86] It also decreases low-grade inflammation (which contributes to insulin resistance and damages the insulin-producing cells of the pancreas).[87] It does this directly by inhibiting pro-inflammatory molecules and indirectly by acting as an antioxidant, reducing cell-damaging free radicals and the associated inflammation.[88] This vital mineral also helps repair damage to the cellular machinery that prepares glucose to be used for energy.[89]

An analysis of seven separate clinical trials totaling nearly 400 Type 2 diabetics found that chromium supplementation in doses ranging from 400 to 1,000 mcg per day was effective at lowering fasting blood sugar levels.[90]

Vanadium, meanwhile, is found in a wide variety of herbs, fruits, and vegetables (such as green beans, carrots, onions, tomatoes, garlic, black pepper, and parsley to name a few) and is thought to reduce blood sugar levels via an insulin-like effect. Low blood levels of vanadium correlate with increased risk for Type 2 diabetes,[91] and in a study of Type 1 diabetics, supplementation with vanadium for 2½ years resulted in a

30% drop in insulin use, and a 36% drop in fasting blood sugar levels, as well as a reduction in total cholesterol.[92] The only adverse side effect reported in this study was some mild diarrhea at the beginning that resolved on its own.

A word of caution: Taking high doses of chromium and vanadium for long periods of time can cause them to accumulate to toxic levels.[93,94,95] It's better to either get these from eating a healthy diet, or else you should consult your healthcare provider for guidance in proper dosage for your individual health needs.

Gymnema

Gymnema sylvestre is an herb long used in traditional Ayurvedic medicine. Its common Indian name, gurmar, means "sugar destroyer," because gymnema contains several compounds that block sweet receptors. What patients notice is that they have far less sugar cravings. This is because the gymnema stabilizes blood sugar. This herb is also used to decrease cholesterol and inflammation, ease digestive ailments, prevent tooth decay, fight free radicals, and even fend off cancer.[96]

In the intestinal tract, gymnema slows the absorption of glucose and fats. Upon entering your bloodstream, it circulates to your pancreas where it promotes the secretion of insulin and helps convert it into its active form.[97] Gymnema also activates enzymes involved in breaking down glucose to produce energy,[98] inhibits release of glucose from the liver into the bloodstream,[99] and promotes repair and regeneration of insulin-producing cells. At the same time as it stimulates glucose burning, gymnema inhibits your body from burning fats for energy. In this way available glucose stores are used preferentially, helping to keep your blood sugar levels within a healthy range. In preliminary studies gymnema has demonstrated the ability to reduce Hemoglobin A1c levels,[100] proof positive of this herb's blood sugar-lowering effects.

As an antioxidant, gymnema protects against the damaging effects that result from chronic high blood sugar levels, such as oxidation of cholesterol. In one preliminary study, gymnema decreased oxidized cholesterol by 31%.[101] Supplementation with gymnema has also been shown to increase levels of antioxidant enzymes.[102]

One safety concern regarding gymnema is whether it might actually lower blood sugar *too* much! Some studies indicate that moderate doses of gymnema may lower blood sugar levels in diabetics, but not in non-diabetics, indicating a high safety profile for this herb.[103] However, high doses of gymnema have been shown to cause hypoglycemia.[104]

Alpha-Lipoic Acid

A fatty acid your body manufactures in small quantities, alpha-lipoic acid, is present in every cell, where it assists in the breakdown of glucose and amino acids to produce energy.[105] Alpha-lipoic acid helps manage blood sugar by making cells more sensitive to insulin, prompting them to absorb glucose and thereby lowering blood sugar levels.[106] In one study, Type 2 diabetics, who took 300 mg of alpha-lipoic acid per day for two months, showed significant decreases in fasting blood sugar, post-meal blood sugar, and insulin levels.[107] Alpha-lipoic acid also calms the body's inflammatory response, which is a major contributing factor to diabetic complications.[108]

Perhaps the most important function of this compound, and the one that has garnered the most attention, is its significant antioxidant benefits. Alpha-lipoic acid regenerates other antioxidants back to their active forms once they've done their work. And in true hero fashion, alpha-lipoic acid may also be capable of stepping in and performing the functions of other antioxidants if their levels become depleted.[109]

Alpha-lipoic acid is further distinguished in that it possesses a structure that is both water-soluble and fat-soluble. This singular characteristic makes it highly versatile and able to function in many parts of your body. Its ability to interact with fats makes it particularly helpful for healing and preventing diabetic peripheral neuropathy. A study of Type 2 diabetics with longstanding symptoms of peripheral neuropathy of the hands and feet showed that alpha-lipoic acid supplementation reduced symptoms by up to 40% within four months of treatment.[110] Some evidence suggests that alpha-lipoic acid supplementation may be even more effective for healing autonomic peripheral neuropathy—nerves to the heart and other internal organs—than it is for healing and protecting nerves to the hands and feet.[111]

Tip: This supplement absorbs up to 30% more effectively when taken on an empty stomach.[112]

Some people might get heartburn taking alpha lipoic acid—if, so, take it with a small snack.

Biotin

Biotin is a water-soluble, B-complex vitamin that assists the enzymes that break down carbohydrates, fats, and proteins into usable energy. It affects blood sugar regulation at the genetic level, improving function of the genes that control insulin production.[113]

While in small quantities, biotin is found in a variety of animal and plant foods, including egg yolk, sardines, legumes, nuts, and whole grains. Your beneficial intestinal bacteria produce biotin, as well. Deficiency of this essential nutrient is rare, but has been associated with low blood sugar and insulin levels and impaired structure of insulin-producing cells.[114] Biotin deficiency also results in increased secretion of glucagon, a hormone that raises blood sugar by depleting the liver's glycogen stores.[115]

Conversely, preliminary studies have demonstrated that supplementing with high levels of biotin increases insulin secretion and may improve the structure and function of pancreas cells.[116] One study demonstrated that insulin-producing cells of biotin-supplemented mice were larger and structurally superior to those of non-supplemented mice.[117] Biotin supplementation may also improve glucose tolerance and lead to more robust insulin production in response to glucose. In diabetic animals, biotin has been shown to decrease post-meal blood sugar spikes.[118] Drug companies have begun experimenting with incorporating biotin into oral insulin medications to improve their effectiveness. Results of one such study showed that biotin-enhanced insulin was absorbed up to five times more efficiently compared to conventional oral insulin drugs.[119]

Biotin has also been found to work synergistically with chromium. Several human clinical trials report reductions in fasting blood sugar and increased insulin sensitivity, as well as decreased cholesterol levels with chromium-biotin supplementation.[120,121,122,123] In one study, the combination reduced Hemoglobin A1c levels in Type 2 diabetics with poorly controlled blood sugar levels by up to 1.9%,[124] putting the nutritional supplement on an equal footing with some of the most commonly prescribed oral diabetes medications.

With no reported side effects at the dosages and treatment durations used, chromium-biotin supplementation may present a superior option in terms of effectiveness.

White Mulberry Leaf Extract

White Mulberry Leaf is highly regarded in both Chinese and Japanese medicine for its effect on blood sugar and blood lipids, and there's research evidence as well for its glucose control. It contains a "sugar-blocker" (specifically alpha-glucosidase inhibitor), which has great blood sugar-lowering effects.

This study showed that, when compared to a placebo, white mulberry lowered blood sugar in diabetics for over 2 hours after eating foods containing sugar.[125] Other studies have shown that, compared to the diabetic drug glyburide, white mulberry dropped blood glucose and Hemoglobin A1c numbers much more effectively. It also has a positive effect on blood lipids.

White mulberry bark also has a positive effect on weight. While this probably comes from having better glucose control and lower blood sugar, this study still showed that, after measuring at 30, 60, and 90 days, the group taking the white mulberry extract had significantly better weight loss than the placebo group.[126]

CONCLUSION

I spent years making a lot of the same mistakes you and many other people have made, and even more years to put this information together in a way that made sense, both to me, and to my patients. I had to redo all my thinking about fats, and about "good carbs," and figure out how exercise fit into this. I had to figure out why some of my patients succeeded and why others didn't, and how to adjust my recommendations. And after years of doing this, the medical establishment is finally starting to catch up—with many of the same recommendations now being suggested by forward-thinking MD's, as well.

But instead of waiting for them (since research is often 10 years ahead of standard medical advice), I've just decided to give this information to you directly, so that you can take control of your own health, and get yourself back on the path to feeling good and being well! Thank you for wanting to take back your health and for allowing me to be a part of that journey.

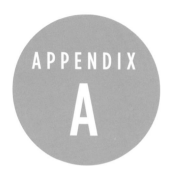

APPENDIX
A

GETTING THE HANG OF EATING HEALTHY

QUICK & EASY TIPS

- Nuts and nut butters make great snacks. Keep them in your purse, gym bag, etc.—they'll feed your brain and then you won't be tempted to go for the chips. Just don't go crazy with them—too much of them aren't healthy either (eating too many nuts is a common mistake, so make sure you have other snacks available as well). The recommended daily serving size of nuts is a ⅓ of a cup, so measure your nuts out initially to see how much that is.

- Keep some guacamole or hummus in the fridge (make sure it's not heavily processed) to eat with carrots, celery sticks, or cucumbers.

- Hard-boil some eggs to keep as a quick snack, or use the whole dozen to make egg salad for a few days.

- Buy (or make your own) beef, turkey, or salmon jerky.

- Use real butter instead of a spread, real bacon instead of turkey bacon, and half-and-half or whole milk instead of low fat or skim.

EASY SUBSTITUTIONS

The following can make great substitutes for your usual carb-dense foods:

- Flavored sparkling water (or sparkling water with a splash of juice or a few drops of flavored stevia) instead of soda

- Spaghetti squash or zucchini noodles instead of pasta (consider getting one of those vegetable spiralizers to make your own)

- Xylitol instead of sugar

- Mashed cauliflower instead mashed potatoes

- Grated cauliflower instead of rice

- Black beans instead of flour

I had a patient who was modifying her diet and realized how addicted to carbs her 13-year old was. Her daughter's favorite dish was a mix of chicken, cheese, and rice, and she adamantly said she "hated" cauliflower. One evening, my patient (the mom), substituted grated cauliflower for the rice, and her daughter not only didn't notice, but her mother was able to keep doing it for months before telling her.

Recently I was visiting a friend who took me to see her sister-in-law, who had been a patient of mine. This patient had made huge changes in her diet and was doing fantastically, and she urged me to try her brownies. The main ingredient was: black beans! I was blown away. We tested it on a guest who came by, and he said "Yum!" *before* we told him it was made from black beans. He said that, if he hadn't tried it first, he'd have never believed it could be that good!

- So before you say, "no way" to these suggestions, (and there are many more on the internet!), give them a try—you might be very pleasantly surprised at how easy it is to find a healthy, low-carb substitution for your favorite food!

6 TIPS FOR DINING OUT

Remember that this is not meant to be a "no-carb" diet. This is designed so that if you'd like to have something that is carb-dense, you just balance it out. The trick to not wrecking your 60 gram allotment is to avoid having a ton of carbs, especially early in the day. If you find yourself wanting to dine out, just follow these tips.

Tip 1: Even if they don't say it on the menu, most restaurants are willing to make substitutions for free, especially vegetables. So if you don't see anything obvious on the menu, just ask. For example, you might be able to exchange the side of rice for a side salad for no cost, or maybe just $1.

Tip 2: As soon as they bring your meal, ask for a to-go box. By packing up half of your meal right away, this will help you avoid overeating, and the leftovers make a quick and easy lunch for the next day.

Tip 3: Split your meal with your dining partner, and get an extra salad to split as well—when you start doing this, you'll quickly notice how disproportionately huge desserts are in restaurants, and you'll wish they would bring you one a quarter the size. You could also get a sandwich, but leave half the bread off. Or, cut the sandwich in half—eat half now, and save the rest for later.

Tip 4: We all love those taco places, and it can be easy to modify food there. If they're making your burrito as you're walking down the line, start with putting it in a bowl. Leave off the rice, get a fraction of the beans, and get extra guacamole plus any other toppings (like pico de gallo), and you're set. Or, if you're in a restaurant, order the fajitas (vegetable or meat), and ask them to not include the rice and beans. Have 1 or 2 tortillas (10 grams of carbs each), and you've had a tasty AND low-carb meal! Remember to order the "skinny margarita" if you want one—they'll leave out the sugary mixes.

Tip 5: Ask for club soda with lime for your drink (maybe even served in a wine glass!), so that you have something special to drink, but it wasn't a soda.

Tip 6: There are some hamburger and sandwich chains now that serve low-carb meals with the hamburger or sandwich fixings wrapped in lettuce. And if they don't offer it on the menu, it never hurts to just ask for it, and see what they can do for you.

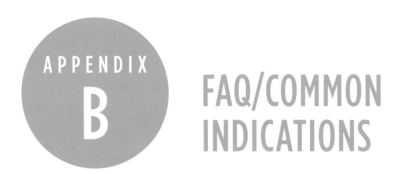

FAQ/COMMON INDICATIONS

Many people notice huge improvements in how they feel, and in their overall health, by controlling their blood sugar. But as with any change in diet or lifestyle, there may be a few issues that come up. This section should answer most of your questions. If your issue persists, or you don't get relief after following our suggestions, please see your physician.

"I am experiencing tiredness and fatigue."

Your body is beginning to generate the enzymes necessary to efficiently burn protein and fat for energy, and it may take one person a little longer than another. Generally, it's about two weeks, depending on how much you restricted carbs in your diet.

Ask yourself these questions, and try these recommendations:

- **Are you eating frequently enough?** Going too long between meals or skipping meals will make you tired. Eat every 2-3 hours.

- **Are you eating enough calories?** We don't encourage calorie counting, but sometimes people cut their carbs and don't replace the calories with protein or fat. Don't be afraid of healthy fats – remember, fats by themselves won't make you fat.

- **Are you drinking enough water?** The estimate is half your bodyweight, in ounces. So if you're 150 pounds, that's 75 ounces of water per day.

- **Are you getting enough sleep?** A minimum of 7-8 hours a night is vital.

Don't over-exercise in this period of time if you're tired, as your body is already trying to make changes, and if you tend to exercise a lot, it might all be a bit too much. Just keep it in moderation until your system has adjusted.

"I have constipation."

Carbohydrates feed the bacteria in your gut that give your stools bulk. But carbs can also irritate your colon and force it to move—masking a weak digestion.

Try these suggestions:

- Drink plenty of water.

- Eat more fibrous vegetables or add a fruit (like an apple) every day or two.

- Try an herbal laxative, like Smooth Move® Tea (available in health food stores).

- Weak stomach acid can also cause digestive problems like constipation. Try adding ½ to 1 teaspoon of apple cider vinegar to your glass of water at mealtimes.

"I have gas and bloating."

Most people notice a big reduction in gas and bloating by reducing carbs, but sometimes they can be caused by other reasons, like weak digestion.

Try these suggestions:

- Make sure you're not eating more carbs than you realize. Sugars and carbs cause a lot of gas, more than people think. You can easily measure the grams of carbs you're eating each by using simple, online tools. These can be found on many websites, such as: www.myfitnesspal.com or www.loseit.com

- Drinking a glass of water with ½ to 1 teaspoon of apple cider vinegar at mealtime will also help with gas and bloating.

"I'm burping a lot and having loose/light-colored stools."

Initially, if you have a weak gallbladder, it may not be able to handle a diet that is higher in fat. Try easing into this a bit more slowly, to get your body used to eating more fat and protein.

- Many natural practitioners can help with gallbladder issues. Try finding one in your area who can help to restore and improve your overall digestive health.

- We strongly recommend contacting your physician if your symptoms are severe or if you have diarrhea lasting longer than 24 hours.

- Make sure you are drinking plenty of water!

"I fell off the wagon, and am eating too many carbs again, and my cravings came back. What should I do?"

First, it's totally normal to fall off that wagon—you're learning a new way of eating and dealing with decades of different habits—so it'll take some practice. All you have to do is get back on the wagon.

It's kind of like this: you have this dragon that's been fed sugar and carbs for a long time. When you were eating low-carb, you put him to sleep. But when you ate that birthday cake (or lasagna, or dessert), you woke him up again. It'll take a little bit to get him to go back to sleep.

When you've been eating low-carb long enough, the dragon eventually goes away. You'll know this, because you might have that birthday cake, but it won't give you cravings again, or wipe you out. So just keep practicing, and continue to get right back on that wagon!

"I exercise a lot—how will this affect me?"

Many athletes are taught to eat carbs—after all, the term "carb-loading" came from them! But many of them have blood sugar problems, evidenced by scores of overweight exercisers, and the coaching they get is to eat something sugar/carb-like every 45 minutes while training. This is probably the biggest falsehood perpetrated against athletes. It is absolutely possible, and actually preferable, to eat low carb. Your energy levels will stay more stable, you'll have more endurance, you'll have much better energy, and it's overall better for your health.

It takes about 2 weeks to get your body used to eating a higher protein/higher fat diet when you're exercising. Initially, you might notice that you're a little more tired, or that you can't exercise as long. That's all normal—think of it like you're converting your car from one that's gas-powered to a more efficient, electric-powered model.

It'll take a little bit to get the conversion to occur, but once you do, it'll be great!

To learn more about being a low-carb athlete, visit Mark Sisson's site: www.marksdailyapple.com. He was a former Ironman (placing fourth in the Hawaii Ironman competition) but struggled with his health. Finally, he learned about low-carb and nutrition. He's a fantastic testament to being a low-carb athlete!

"I've just started eating healthier, and I'm having terrible headaches."

Sugar and carbs are addictive, and your body is letting you know that. You're going through a detox, so make sure you're drinking enough water. Ease into this way of eating a little slower if that's what feels right. And if you need to, take an over-the-counter pain medication once or twice. It should clear up in a day or so.

"My weight loss is stuck."

Our experience has shown that, even with the guidelines of 60 grams of carbs per day, some people get "stuck". Common places where individuals may have problems can be:

Eating Too Much Fruit, Not Enough Veggies: Some people can handle more than others, so make sure you're not eating too much. Our general guidelines are to eat at least twice as many vegetables as fruit.

Over-Snacking on Nuts: It's easy to overeat nuts, and at some point, calories DO count, so watch how much you eat, and check the carb count on your nuts. For example, cashews (so many people's favorite!), are the highest in carbs compared to other nuts. So just pay attention.

Misjudging Alcohol Intake: You might have the numbers right regarding the carb counts, but alcohol metabolizes differently, and in some people, will prevent weight loss or even cause weight gain. Like I mentioned earlier, a gram of carbs has 4 calories, and a gram of fat has 9 calories, but a gram of alcohol has 7. And those liquid calories go down very easily. Try reducing your alcohol intake and see what happens.

Not eating enough, or frequently enough: Some people might be eating low-carb, but simply aren't getting enough calories. Make sure your breakfast is substantial, and that you actually eat an adequate amount of calories throughout your day. Not eating enough calories will slow your metabolism, preventing weight loss.

Not Getting Enough Exercise: While it's possible to lose weight by making simple, dietary changes, it goes much faster if you're also exercising. I would even say that, unless you are including some exercise every day, it would be next-to-impossible to regain health. So please, make this a priority.

Not Getting Enough Sleep: Studies have shown that less than 7 hours of sleep can absolutely inhibit weight loss, make sure you're going to bed early enough!

Not Managing Stress: We've learned that stress causes a lot of problems, and inhibiting weight loss is just one of them. So use the techniques we mentioned to help you lower your stress levels.

Of course, other things may be affecting weight loss as well. Thyroid function, adrenal function, and your body's ability to clear estrogen will all affect weight loss. You may need to find someone to help you with these issues, and natural practitioners—like certified nutritionists, naturopathic doctors, acupuncturists, and doctors trained in functional medicine—can all help.

"I've been eating low carb, but my blood sugar numbers aren't coming down."

Has this happened to you? You're eating really well, but your fasting blood sugar numbers in the morning continue to be high. It seems so unfair, right? This is where I have to explain to people that getting healthy is sometimes not a clear "cause-and-effect". Just because you're "behaving" at this moment doesn't mean your body will always be able to instantly be well. Let me explain.

One of the ways a body starts to "break" when it has high blood sugar is it starts to store those excess calories in the liver. Then, for weeks, sometimes months after you've started eating healthy, your liver continues to dump out glucose into the bloodstream, especially at night. This results in the higher blood sugar numbers in the morning.

The one thing you *can* do in the immediate sense is exercise to get the glucose out of the bloodstream. So exercising first thing, like those short quick intense exercises I mentioned earlier, can be hugely helpful. Another action to take is to do those exercise "snacks" I wrote about earlier—doing some late in the day can help your blood sugar at night and therefore in the morning. And just keep going with your new way of eating. At some point, the liver will be "empty," and your numbers will be normal again. Don't give up!

"How long does it take to reverse my diabetes?"

It depends on how long you've had the disease, and how much damage has occurred. Some people will notice that their blood sugar numbers start dropping within a short time, and others can take longer. Sometimes, blood sugar numbers won't drop for a while because the body has too much insulin resistance, which makes it vital to stick to this program to keep insulin out of the system and re-sensitize the insulin receptor sites on the cells. Doing the short, intense-style exercise will speed this up.

Reducing the glucose (and therefore the insulin) in your body is the most pivotal part of turning this disease around.

You may need to stay on your medication for a while—just keep monitoring your blood glucose, and keep your doctor updated.

Typically, the average is 12 to 18 months if someone has diabetes, and usually less if they have insulin resistance. It just depends on how much you adhere to this. I've had patients who couldn't get blood test numbers to change until they did the exercise "snacks" (on page 65) even though they were already exercising. I've had other patients who had to eat less than 60 grams of carbs to cause a change...and others who couldn't do carbs at dinner at all. Still others who took longer (but never gave up!) or who needed, at some point, to deal with calories, or even others who had bariatric surgery but then STILL kept going on making good choices!

Maybe you know someone who had one of these surgeries. Or you've contemplated it yourself, and are wondering about the pros and cons?

One of the definite pros is that it almost instantly reverses diabetes. Along with reversing diabetes, all sorts of other health markers improve, including cardiovascular markers, and even improving your gut bacteria! And, of course, there's the weight loss, which typically continues for up to 2 years.

The downsides are: it's a surgery, and surgeries have risks, including death. There's the issue of malnutrition—like I mentioned earlier, most people have subclinical malnutrition, and they're eating normal portions. What happens when people eat very little? Their malnourishment gets worse.

Then there's the weight gain. Yes, people will lose weight— but statistically most of them gain it back, often because they've never really learned how to eat properly. One of the standard recommendations is to eat low fat and we know how THAT goes! But if people could eat real food, and lower carb, they would keep the weight off.

Interestingly, though, unlike the Biggest Loser™ contestants whose metabolisms were still slow after 6 years, people with bariatric surgeries typically get their normal metabolism back after a year.[127,128]

Just something to keep in mind if this is an issue for you.

Everyone's physiology is different to some degree, so some personal modifications may need to happen. But it still comes down to this:

There are NO OTHER OPTIONS to reversing diabetes and insulin resistance. Not by eating "healthy, whole-grain carbs", not by eating low fat, not by taking insulin (like I mentioned before, insulin just by itself causes a whole range of serious problems).

In your hands you hold the tools to preventing and reversing many of the major diseases that afflict people these days, and cause our degenerative decline in health as we age. We are thrilled you have taken on your health, and honored that you have allowed us to contribute.

ENDNOTES

Image(s) used under license from Shutterstock.com.

Justin's® is a registered trademark of JUSTIN'S, LLC

TRUVIA® is a registered trademark of Cargill, Incorporated

Pure Via® is a registered trademark of Whole Earth Sweetener Company LLC

MyFitnessPal.com® is a registered trademark of Under Armour, Inc.

LoseIt!® is a registered trademark of FitNow, Inc.

Smooth Move® is a registered trademark of Traditional Medicinals®

The Biggest Loser® is a trademark of Reveille LLC and its related entities.

Joel Silver, *The Matrix*, Film, Keanu Reeves, Laurence Fishburne (1999; Warner Bros. Studio).

REFERENCES

1. American Diabetes Association. "Statistics About Diabetes." *American Diabetes Association.* Accessed November 21, 2016. http://www.diabetes.org/diabetes-basics/statistics/.

2. "About Diabetes." *Congressional Diabetes Caucus,* August 6, 2014. https://diabetescaucus-degette.house.gov/facts-and-figures.

3. DiNicolantonio, James J., and Sean C. Lucan. "The Wrong White Crystals: Not Salt but Sugar as Aetiological in Hypertension and Cardiometabolic Disease." *Open Heart 1,* no. 1 (November 1, 2014): e000167. doi:10.1136/openhrt-2014-000167.

4. Garg, Rajesh, Gordon H. Williams, Shelley Hurwitz, et al. "Low-Salt Diet Increases Insulin Resistance in Healthy Subjects." *Metabolism - Clinical and Experimental* 60, no. 7 (July 2011): 965–68. doi:10.1016/j.metabol.2010.09.005.

5. Yager, James D., and Nancy E. Davidson. "Estrogen Carcinogenesis in Breast Cancer." *The New England Journal of Medicine* 354, no. 3 (January 19, 2006): 270–82. doi:10.1056/NEJMra050776.

6. Beral, Valerie, Diana Bull, Gillian Reeves, and Million Women Study Collaborators. "Endometrial Cancer and Hormone-Replacement Therapy in the Million Women Study." *Lancet* 365, no. 9470 (May 30, 2005): 1543–51. doi: 10.1016/S0140-6736(05)66455-0.

7. Carruba, Giuseppe. "Estrogen and Prostate Cancer: An Eclipsed Truth in an Androgen-Dominated Scenario." *Journal of Cellular Biochemistry* 102, no. 4 (November 1, 2007): 899–911. doi:10.1002/jcb.21529.

8. "How Diabetes Drives Atherosclerosis." *ScienceDaily.* Accessed November 21, 2016. https://www.sciencedaily.com/releases/2008/03/080313124430.htm.

9. Quiñones-Galvan, A., A. M. Sironi, S. Baldi, et al. "Evidence That Acute Insulin Administration Enhances LDL Cholesterol Susceptibility to Oxidation in Healthy Humans." *Arteriosclerosis, Thrombosis, and Vascular Biology* 19, no. 12 (December 1999): 2928–32. PMID: 10591671.

10. Loon, B. J. Potter van, C. Kluft, J. K. Radder, et al. "The Cardiovascular Risk Factor Plasminogen Activator Inhibitor Type 1 Is Related to Insulin Resistance." *Metabolism* 42, no. 8 (August 1, 1993): 945–49. doi:10.1016/0026-0495(93)90005-9.

11. American Diabetes Association. "Statistics About Diabetes." *American Diabetes Association.* Accessed November 21, 2016. http://www.diabetes.org/diabetes-basics/statistics/.

12. Monte, Suzanne M. de la, and Jack R. Wands. "Alzheimer's Disease Is Type 3 Diabetes–Evidence Reviewed." *Journal of Diabetes Science and Technology* 2, no. 6 (November 2008): 1101–13. doi: 10.1177/193229680800200619.

13. Wilbert, Caroline. "Diabetes Can Double Odds of Alzheimer's." *WebMD.* Accessed November 21, 2016. http://www.webmd.com/diabetes/news/20090130/diabetes-can-double-odds-of-alzheimers.

14. Taubes, Gary. "Is Sugar Toxic?" *The New York Times,* April 13, 2011. http://www.nytimes.com/2011/04/17/magazine/mag-17Sugar-t.html.

15. Apple, Sam. "An Old Idea, Revived: Starve Cancer to Death." *The New York Times,* May 12, 2016. http://www.nytimes.com/2016/05/15/magazine/warburg-effect-an-old-idea-revived-starve-cancer-to-death.html.

16. Anderson, R. J., K. E. Freedland, R. E. Clouse, and P. J. Lustman. "The Prevalence of Comorbid Depression in Adults with Diabetes: A Meta-Analysis." *Diabetes Care* 24, no. 6 (June 2001): 1069–78. doi: 10.2337/diacare.24.6.1069.

17. "Sugar and Your Immune System." *Alternative Health Atlanta,* July 6, 2012. http://alternativehealthatlanta.com/immune-system/sugar-and-your-immune-system/.

18. Westman, Eric C., William S. Yancy, and Margaret Humphreys. "Dietary Treatment of Diabetes Mellitus in the Pre-Insulin Era (1914-1922)." *Perspectives in Biology and Medicine* 49, no. 1 (2006): 77–83. doi: 10.1353/pbm.2006.0017.

19. Sacks, Frank M., Vincent J. Carey, Cheryl A. M. Anderson, et al. "Effects of High vs Low Glycemic Index of Dietary Carbohydrate on Cardiovascular Disease Risk Factors and Insulin Sensitivity: The OmniCarb Randomized Clinical Trial." *JAMA* 312, no. 23 (December 17, 2014): 2531–41. doi: 10.1001/jama.2014.16658.

20. National Institute of Diabetes and Digestive and Kidney Diseases (NIDDK). "Health Statistics." Accessed December 13, 2016. https://www.niddk.nih.gov/health-information/health-statistics/Pages/default.aspx.

21. Bowker, Samantha L., Sumit R. Majumdar, Paul Veugelers, and Jeffrey A. Johnson. "Increased Cancer-Related Mortality for Patients with Type 2 Diabetes Who Use Sulfonylureas or Insulin." *Diabetes Care* 29, no. 2 (February 2006): 254–58. doi: 10.2337/dc06-0997.

22. Donadon, Valter, Massimiliano Balbi, Michela Ghersetti, et al. "Antidiabetic Therapy and Increased Risk of Hepatocellular Carcinoma in Chronic Liver Disease." *World Journal of Gastroenterology* 15, no. 20 (May 28, 2009): 2506–11. PMID: 19469001.

23. Li, Donghui, Sai-Ching J. Yeung, Manal M. Hassan, et al. "Antidiabetic Therapies Affect Risk of Pancreatic Cancer." *Gastroenterology* 137, no. 2 (August 2009): 482–88. doi: 10.1053/j.gastro.2009.04.013.

24. Lebovitz, Harold E. "Insulin: Potential Negative Consequences of Early Routine Use in Patients With Type 2 Diabetes." *Diabetes Care* 34, Supplement 2 (May 1, 2011): S225–30. doi: 10.2337/dc11-s225.

25. Henry, R. R., B. Gumbiner, T. Ditzler, et al. "Intensive Conventional Insulin Therapy for Type II Diabetes. Metabolic Effects during a 6-Mo Outpatient Trial." *Diabetes Care* 16, no. 1 (January 1993): 21–31.

26. Purnell, J. Q., J. E. Hokanson, S. M. Marcovina, et al. "Effect of Excessive Weight Gain with Intensive Therapy of Type 1 Diabetes on Lipid Levels and Blood Pressure: Results from the DCCT. Diabetes Control and Complications Trial." *JAMA* 280, no. 2 (July 8, 1998): 140–46. doi: 10.2337/diacare.16.1.21.

27. Inzucchi, Silvio E., Frederick A. Masoudi, Yongfei Wang, et al. "Insulin-Sensitizing Antihyperglycemic Drugs and Mortality after Acute Myocardial Infarction: Insights from the National Heart Care Project." *Diabetes Care* 28, no. 7 (July 2005): 1680–89. doi: 10.2337/diacare.28.7.1680.

28. Westman, Eric C., William S. Yancy, and Margaret Humphreys. "Dietary Treatment of Diabetes Mellitus in the Pre-Insulin Era (1914-1922)." *Perspectives in Biology and Medicine* 49, no. 1 (2006): 77–83. doi: 10.1353/pbm.2006.0017.

29. Frye, R. L., P. August, M. M. Brooks, et al. "A Randomized Trial of Therapies for Type 2 Diabetes and Coronary Artery Disease." *New England Journal of Medicine* 360, no. 24 (June 11, 2009): 2503–15. doi: 10.1056/NEJMoa0805796.

30. Light, Luise. "A Fatally Flawed Food Guide." Accessed December 13, 2016. http://www.whale.to/a/light.html.

31. Light, Luise. *What to Eat: The Ten Things You Really Need to Know to Eat Well and Be Healthy*. 1 edition. New York: McGraw-Hill Education, 2006. https://books.google.com/books/about/What_to_Eat.html?id=Gjx7OI7i-P8C.

32. Bremer, Andrew A., Michele Mietus-Snyder, and Robert H. Lustig. "Toward a Unifying Hypothesis of Metabolic Syndrome." *Pediatrics* 129, no. 3 (March 2012): 557–70. doi: 10.1542/peds.2011-2912.

33. Volkow, Nora D., et al. "Neurobiologic Advances from the Brain Disease Model of Addiction." *New England Journal of Medicine* 374, no. 4 (January 28, 2016): 363-371. doi: org/10.1056/NEJMra1511480

33. Hu, T., L. Yao, K. Reynolds, et al. "Adherence to Low-Carbohydrate and Low-Fat Diets in Relation to Weight Loss and Cardiovascular Risk Factors." *Obesity Science & Practice* 2, no. 1 (March 1, 2016): 24–31. doi: 10.1002/osp4.23.

34. Ebbeling, Cara B., Janis F. Swain, Henry A. Feldman, et al. "Effects of Dietary Composition on Energy Expenditure During Weight-Loss Maintenance." *JAMA* 307, no. 24 (June 27, 2012): 2627–34. doi: 10.1001/jama.2012.6607.

35. Fothergill, Erin, Juen Guo, Lilian Howard, et al. "Persistent Metabolic Adaptation 6 Years after 'The Biggest Loser' Competition." *Obesity* 24, no. 8 (August 1, 2016): 1612–19. doi: 10.1002/oby.21538.

36. Ames, Bruce N. "Low Micronutrient Intake May Accelerate the Degenerative Diseases of Aging through Allocation of Scarce Micronutrients by Triage." *Proceedings of the National Academy of Sciences of the United States of America* 103, no. 47 (November 21, 2006): 17589–94. doi: 10.1073/pnas.0608757103.

37. McCann, Joyce C., and Bruce N. Ames. "Adaptive Dysfunction of Selenoproteins from the Perspective of the Triage Theory: Why Modest Selenium Deficiency May Increase Risk of Diseases of Aging." *The FASEB Journal* 25, no. 6 (June 2011): 1793–1814. doi: 10.1096/fj.11-180885.

38. McCann, Joyce C., and Bruce N. Ames. "Vitamin K, an Example of Triage Theory: Is Micronutrient Inadequacy Linked to Diseases of Aging?" *The American Journal of Clinical Nutrition* 90, no. 4 (October 2009): 889–907. doi: 10.3945/ajcn.2009.27930.

39. Kaidar-Person, Orit, Benjamin Person, Samuel Szomstein, and Raul J. Rosenthal. "Nutritional Deficiencies in Morbidly Obese Patients: A New Form of Malnutrition? Part A: Vitamins." *Obesity Surgery* 18, no. 7 (July 2008): 870–76. doi: 10.1007/s11695-007-9349-y.

40. Jager, Jolien de, Adriaan Kooy, Philippe Lehert, et al. "Long Term Treatment with Metformin in Patients with Type 2 Diabetes and Risk of Vitamin B-12 Deficiency: Randomised Placebo Controlled Trial." *The BMJ* 340 (May 20, 2010): c2181. doi: 10.2307/40702163.

41. Ting, Rose Zhao-Wei, Cheuk Chun Szeto, Michael Ho-Ming Chan, et al. "Risk Factors of Vitamin B(12) Deficiency in Patients Receiving Metformin." *Archives of Internal Medicine* 166, no. 18 (October 9, 2006): 1975–79. doi: 10.1001/archinte.166.18.1975.

42. Taubes, Gary. "What If It's All Been a Big Fat Lie?" *The New York Times*, July 7, 2002. http://www.nytimes.com/2002/07/07/magazine/what-if-it-s-all-been-a-big-fat-lie.html.

43. Walsh, Bryan. "Ending the War on Fat." *Time Magazine* 183, no. 24 (June 23, 2014): 28-35. http://time.com/vault/issue/2014-06-23/page/31/.

44. "Lard: The New Health Food?" *Food & Wine*. Accessed November 21, 2016. http://www.foodandwine.com/articles/lard-the-new-health-food.

45. Lustig, Robert H. "Fructose: It's 'Alcohol Without the Buzz.'" *Advances in Nutrition: An International Review Journal* 4, no. 2 (March 1, 2013): 226–35. doi: 10.3945/an.112.002998.

46. Wanless, I. R., and J. S. Lentz. "Fatty Liver Hepatitis (Steatohepatitis) and Obesity: An Autopsy Study with Analysis of Risk Factors." *Hepatology* 12, no. 5 (November 1990): 1106–10. doi: 10.1002/hep.1840120505.

47. Stanhope, Kimber L., Andrew A. Bremer, Valentina Medici, et al. "Consumption of Fructose and High Fructose Corn Syrup Increase Postprandial Triglycerides, LDL-Cholesterol, and Apolipoprotein-B in Young Men and Women." *The Journal of Clinical Endocrinology and Metabolism* 96, no. 10 (October 2011): E1596-1605. doi: 10.1210/jc.2011-1251.

48. Wei, Yuren, Dong Wang, Gretchen Moran, et al. "Fructose-Induced Stress Signaling in the Liver Involves Methylglyoxal." *Nutrition & Metabolism* 10 (April 8, 2013): 32. doi: 10.1186/1743-7075-10-32.

49. Elliott, Sharon S., Nancy L. Keim, Judith S. Stern, et al. "Fructose, Weight Gain, and the Insulin Resistance Syndrome." *The American Journal of Clinical Nutrition* 76, no. 5 (November 1, 2002): 911–22. doi: 10.1186/1743-7075-2-5.

50. *Ibid.*

51. Mathur, Abhishek, Megan Marine, Debao Lu, et al. "Nonalcoholic Fatty Pancreas Disease." *HPB* 9, no. 4 (2007): 312–18. doi: 10.1080/13651820701504157.

52. Geenen, Erwin-Jan M. van, Mark M. Smits, Tim C. M. A. Schreuder, et al. "Nonalcoholic Fatty Liver Disease Is Related to Nonalcoholic Fatty Pancreas Disease." *Pancreas* 39, no. 8 (November 2010): 1185–90. doi: 10.1097/MPA.0b013e3181f6fce2.

53. Szczepaniak, Lidia S., Ronald G. Victor, Lelio Orci, and Roger H. Unger. "Forgotten but Not Gone: The Rediscovery of Fatty Heart, the Most Common Unrecognized Disease in America." *Circulation Research* 101, no. 8 (October 12, 2007): 759–67. doi: 10.1161/CIRCRESAHA.107.160457.

54. Guzzardi, Maria A., and Patricia Iozzo. "Fatty Heart, Cardiac Damage, and Inflammation." *The Review of Diabetic Studies* 8, no. 3 (2011): 403–17. doi: 10.1900/RDS.2011.8.403.

55. Leite, Nathalie C., Gil F. Salles, Antonio L. E. Araujo, et al. "Prevalence and Associated Factors of Non-Alcoholic Fatty Liver Disease in Patients with Type-2 Diabetes Mellitus." *Liver International* 29, no. 1 (January 2009): 113–19. doi: 10.1111/j.1478-3231.2008.01718.x.

56. *Ibid.*

57. Allan, Christian B., and Wolfgang Lutz. *Life Without Bread: How a Low-Carbohydrate Diet Can Save Your Life.* 1 edition. Los Angeles, CA: McGraw-Hill Education, 2000. https://books.google.com/books/about/Life_Without_Bread.html?id=NJ6oNV3q3X0C.

58. Westman, Eric C., William S. Yancy, and Margaret Humphreys. "Dietary Treatment of Diabetes Mellitus in the Pre-Insulin Era (1914-1922)." *Perspectives in Biology and Medicine* 49, no. 1 (2006): 77–83. doi: 10.1353/pbm.2006.0017.

59. Félétou, Michel, and Paul M. Vanhoutte. "Endothelial Dysfunction: A Multifaceted Disorder (The Wiggers Award Lecture)." *American Journal of Physiology* 291, no. 3 (September 2006): H985-1002. doi: 10.1152/ajpheart.00292.2006.

60. Pinkney, J. H., C. D. Stehouwer, S. W. Coppack, and J. S. Yudkin. "Endothelial Dysfunction: Cause of the Insulin Resistance Syndrome." *Diabetes* 46, Supplement 2 (September 1997): S9-13. http://dx.doi.org/10.2337/diab.46.2.S9.

61. Kennedy, J. W., M. F. Hirshman, E. V. Gervino, et al. "Acute Exercise Induces GLUT4 Translocation in Skeletal Muscle of Normal Human Subjects and Subjects with Type 2 Diabetes." *Diabetes* 48, no. 5 (May 1999): 1192–97. doi: 10.2337/diabetes.48.5.1192.

62. Alibegovic, Amra C., Lise Højbjerre, Mette P. Sonne, et al. "Impact of 9 Days of Bed Rest on Hepatic and Peripheral Insulin Action, Insulin Secretion, and Whole-Body Lipolysis in Healthy Young Male Offspring of Patients With Type 2 Diabetes." *Diabetes* 58, no. 12 (December 1, 2009): 2749–56. doi: 10.2337/db09-0369.

63. Francois, Monique E., James C. Baldi, Patrick J. Manning, et al. "'Exercise Snacks' before Meals: A Novel Strategy to Improve Glycaemic Control in Individuals with Insulin Resistance." *Diabetologia* 57, no. 7 (July 2014): 1437–45. doi: 10.1007/s00125-014-3244-6.

64. Reynolds, Gretchen. "The Scientific 7-Minute Workout." *Well*. http://well.blogs.nytimes.com/2013/05/09/the-scientific-7-minute-workout/.

65. Gliemann, Lasse, Thomas P. Gunnarsson, Ylva Hellsten, and Jens Bangsbo. "10-20-30 Training Increases Performance and Lowers Blood Pressure and VEGF in Runners." *Scandinavian Journal of Medicine & Science in Sports* 25, no. 5 (October 2015): e479-489. doi: 10.1111/sms.12356.

66. Gillen, Jenna B., Brian J. Martin, Martin J. MacInnis, et al. "Twelve Weeks of Sprint Interval Training Improves Indices of Cardiometabolic Health Similar to Traditional Endurance Training despite a Five-Fold Lower Exercise Volume and Time Commitment." *PLOS ONE* 11, no. 4 (April 26, 2016): e0154075. doi: 10.1371/journal.pone.0154075.

67. Brandhorst, Sebastian, and Valter D. Longo. "Fasting and Caloric Restriction in Cancer Prevention and Treatment." In *Metabolism in Cancer*, edited by Thorsten Cramer and Clemens A. Schmitt, 241–66. Recent Results in Cancer Research 207. Springer International Publishing, 2016. doi: 10.1007/978-3-319-42118-6_12.

68. Lee, Changhan, and Valter Longo. "Dietary Restriction with and without Caloric Restriction for Healthy Aging." *F1000Research* 5 (January 29, 2016). doi: 10.12688/f1000research.7136.1.

69. Lettieri, Barbato Daniele, and Katia Aquilano. "Feast and Famine: Adipose Tissue Adaptations for Healthy Aging." *Ageing Research Reviews* 28 (July 2016): 85–93. doi: 10.1016/j.arr.2016.05.007.

70. Brandhorst, Sebastian, Gerardo Navarrete, Min Wei, et al. "Abstract 4313: Periodic Fasting Mimicking Diet Delays Cancer Development and Progression." *Cancer Research* 76, no. 14 Supplement (July 15, 2016): 4313–4313. doi: 10.1158/1538-7445.AM2016-4313.

71. Francois, Monique E., James C. Baldi, Patrick J. Manning, et al. "'Exercise Snacks' before Meals: A Novel Strategy to Improve Glycaemic Control in Individuals with Insulin Resistance." *Diabetologia* 57, no. 7 (July 2014): 1437–45. doi: 10.1007/s00125-014-3244-6.

72. Seton-Rogers, Sarah. "Chemotherapy: Putting Tumours on a Diet." *Nature Reviews Cancer* 16, no. 9 (September 2016): 549–549. doi: 10.1038/nrc.2016.90.

73. Di Biase, Stefano, Changhan Lee, Sebastian Brandhorst, et al. "Fasting-Mimicking Diet Reduces HO-1 to Promote T Cell-Mediated Tumor Cytotoxicity." *Cancer Cell* 30, no. 1 (July 11, 2016): 136–46. doi:10.1016/j.ccell.2016.06.005.

74. Bredesen, Dale E., Edwin C. Amos, Jonathan Canick, et al. "Reversal of Cognitive Decline in Alzheimer's Disease." *Aging* 8, no. 6 (June 2016): 1250–58. doi: 10.18632/aging.100981.

75. Kandimalla, Ramesh, Vani Thirumala, and P. Hemachandra Reddy. "Is Alzheimer's Disease a Type 3 Diabetes? A Critical Appraisal." *Biochimica Et Biophysica Acta*, August 25, 2016. doi: 10.1016/j.bbadis.2016.08.018.

76. Klein, Guy, Jaekyung Kim, Klaus Himmeldirk, et al. "Antidiabetes and Anti-Obesity Activity of Lagerstroemia Speciosa." *Evidence-Based Complementary and Alternative Medicine: eCAM* 4, no. 4 (December 2007): 401–7. doi: 10.1093/ecam/nem013.

77. Takagi, Satoshi, Toshihiro Miura, Chinami Ishibashi, et al. "Effect of Corosolic Acid on the Hydrolysis of Disaccharides." *Journal of Nutritional Science and Vitaminology* 54, no. 3 (June 2008): 266–68. doi: 10.3177/jnsv.54.266.

78. *Ibid.*

79. Stohs, Sidney J., Howard Miller, and Gilbert R. Kaats. "A Review of the Efficacy and Safety of Banaba (Lagerstroemia Speciosa L.) and Corosolic Acid." *Phytotherapy Research* 26, no. 3 (March 2012): 317–24. doi: 10.1002/ptr.3664.

80. Klein, Guy, Jaekyung Kim, Klaus Himmeldirk, et al. "Antidiabetes and Anti-Obesity Activity of Lagerstroemia Speciosa." *Evidence-Based Complementary and Alternative Medicine* 4, no. 4 (December 2007): 401–7. doi: 10.1093/ecam/nem013.

81. Stohs, Sidney J., Howard Miller, and Gilbert R. Kaats. "A Review of the Efficacy and Safety of Banaba (Lagerstroemia Speciosa L.) and Corosolic Acid." *Phytotherapy Research* 26, no. 3 (March 2012): 317–24. doi: 10.1002/ptr.3664.

82. Miura, Toshihiro, Satoshi Takagi, and Torao Ishida. "Management of Diabetes and Its Complications with Banaba (Lagerstroemia Speciosa L.) and Corosolic Acid." *Evidence-Based Complementary and Alternative Medicine* 2012 (2012): 871495. doi: 10.1155/2012/871495.

83. Judy, William V., Siva P. Hari, W. W. Stogsdill, et al. "Antidiabetic Activity of a Standardized Extract (Glucosol™) from Lagerstroemia Speciosa Leaves in Type II Diabetics: A Dose-Dependence Study." *Journal of Ethnopharmacology* 87, no. 1 (July 2003): 115–17. doi: 10.1016/S0378-8741(03)00122-3.

84. Miura, Toshihiro, Satoshi Takagi, and Torao Ishida. "Management of Diabetes and Its Complications with Banaba (Lagerstroemia Speciosa L.) and Corosolic Acid." *Evidence-Based Complementary and Alternative Medicine* 2012 (2012): 871495. doi: 10.1155/2012/871495.

85. *Ibid.*

86. Hua, Yinan, Suzanne Clark, Jun Ren, and Nair Sreejayan. "Molecular Mechanisms of Chromium in Alleviating Insulin Resistance." *The Journal of Nutritional Biochemistry* 23, no. 4 (April 2012): 313–19. doi: 10.1016/j.jnutbio.2011.11.001.

87. Chen, Yen-Lin, Jiunn-Diann Lin, Te-Lin Hsia, et al. "The Effect of Chromium on Inflammatory Markers, 1st and 2nd Phase Insulin Secretion in Type 2 Diabetes." *European Journal of Nutrition* 53, no. 1 (February 2014): 127–33. doi: 10.1007/s00394-013-0508-8.

88. Hua, Yinan, Suzanne Clark, Jun Ren, and Nair Sreejayan. "Molecular Mechanisms of Chromium in Alleviating Insulin Resistance." *The Journal of Nutritional Biochemistry* 23, no. 4 (April 2012): 313–19. doi:10.1016/j.jnutbio.2011.11.001.

89. *Ibid.*

90. Abdollahi, Mohammad, Amir Farshchi, Shekoufeh Nikfar, and Meysam Seyedifar. "Effect of Chromium on Glucose and Lipid Profiles in Patients with Type 2 Diabetes; a Meta-Analysis Review of Randomized Trials." *Journal of Pharmacy & Pharmaceutical Sciences* 16, no. 1 (2013): 99–114. doi: 10.18433/J3G022.

91. Wang, Xia, Taoping Sun, Jun Liu, et al. "Inverse Association of Plasma Vanadium Levels with Newly Diagnosed Type 2 Diabetes in a Chinese Population." *American Journal of Epidemiology* 180, no. 4 (August 15, 2014): 378–84. doi: 10.1093/aje/kwu148.

92. Soveid, Mahmood, Gholam Abbas Dehghani, and Gholamhossein Ranjbar Omrani. "Long-Term Efficacy and Safety of Vanadium in the Treatment of Type 1 Diabetes." *Archives of Iranian Medicine* 16, no. 7 (July 2013): 408–11. doi: 013167/AIM.009.

93. "Office of Dietary Supplements - Dietary Supplement Fact Sheet: Chromium." Accessed November 21, 2016. https://ods.od.nih.gov/factsheets/Chromium-HealthProfessional/.

94. Gruzewska, K., A. Michno, T. Pawelczyk, and H. Bielarczyk. "Essentiality and Toxicity of Vanadium Supplements in Health and Pathology." *Journal of Physiology and Pharmacology* 65, no. 5 (October 2014): 603–11. PMID: 25371519.

95. Preet, Anju, Bihari L. Gupta, Pramod K. Yadava, and Najma Z. Baquer. "Efficacy of Lower Doses of Vanadium in Restoring Altered Glucose Metabolism and Antioxidant Status in Diabetic Rat Lenses." *Journal of Biosciences* 30, no. 2 (March 2005): 221–30. PMID: 15886458.

96. Tiwari, Pragya, B. N. Mishra, and Neelam S. Sangwan. "Phytochemical and Pharmacological Properties of Gymnema Sylvestre: An Important Medicinal Plant." *BioMed Research International* 2014 (2014): 830285. doi: 10.1155/2014/830285.

97. Al-Romaiyan, A., B. Liu, H. Asare-Anane, et al. "A Novel Gymnema Sylvestre Extract Stimulates Insulin Secretion from Human Islets in Vivo and in Vitro." *Phytotherapy Research* 24, no. 9 (September 2010): 1370–76. doi: 10.1002/ptr.3125.

98. Fabio, Giovanni Di, Valeria Romanucci, Anna De Marco, and Armando Zarrelli. "Triterpenoids from Gymnema Sylvestre and Their Pharmacological Activities." *Molecules* 19, no. 8 (June 28, 2014). doi: 10.3390/molecules190810956.

99. Al-Romaiyan, A., B. Liu, H. Asare-Anane, et al. "A Novel Gymnema Sylvestre Extract Stimulates Insulin Secretion from Human Islets in Vivo and in Vitro." *Phytotherapy Research* 24, no. 9 (September 2010): 1370–76. doi: 10.1002/ptr.3125.

100. Fabio, Giovanni Di, Valeria Romanucci, Anna De Marco, and Armando Zarrelli. "Triterpenoids from Gymnema Sylvestre and Their Pharmacological Activities." *Molecules* 19, no. 8 (June 28, 2014). doi: 10.3390/molecules190810956.

101. Kang, Myung-Hwa, Min Sun Lee, Mi-Kyeong Choi, et al. "Hypoglycemic Activity of Gymnema Sylvestre Extracts on Oxidative Stress and Antioxidant Status in Diabetic Rats." *Journal of Agricultural and Food Chemistry* 60, no. 10 (March 14, 2012): 2517–24. doi: 10.1021/jf205086b.

102. Kumar, Vinay, Uma Bhandari, Chakra Dhar Tripathi, and Geetika Khanna. "Evaluation of Antiobesity and Cardioprotective Effect of Gymnema Sylvestre Extract in Murine Model." *Indian Journal of Pharmacology* 44, no. 5 (October 2012): 607–13. doi: 10.4103/0253-7613.100387.

103. Tiwari, Pragya, B. N. Mishra, and Neelam S. Sangwan. "Phytochemical and Pharmacological Properties of Gymnema Sylvestre: An Important Medicinal Plant." *BioMed Research International* 2014 (2014): 830285. doi: 10.1155/2014/830285.

104. Yadav, Mukesh, Amita Lavania, Radha Tomar, et al. "Complementary and Comparative Study on Hypoglycemic and Antihyperglycemic Activity of Various Extracts of Eugenia Jambolana Seed, Momordica Charantia Fruits, Gymnema Sylvestre, and Trigonella Foenum Graecum Seeds in Rats." *Applied Biochemistry and Biotechnology* 160, no. 8 (April 2010): 2388–2400. doi: 10.1007/s12010-009-8799-1.

105. Shay, Kate Petersen, Régis F. Moreau, Eric J. Smith, et al. "Alpha-Lipoic Acid as a Dietary Supplement: Molecular Mechanisms and Therapeutic Potential." *Biochimica et Biophysica Acta* 1790, no. 10 (October 2009): 1149–60. doi: 10.1016/j.bbagen.2009.07.026.

106. "Lipoic Acid." *Linus Pauling Institute,* April 28, 2014. http://lpi.oregonstate.edu/mic/dietary-factors/lipoic-acid.

107. Ansar, Hasti, Zohreh Mazloom, Fatemeh Kazemi, and Najmeh Hejazi. "Effect of Alpha-Lipoic Acid on Blood Glucose, Insulin Resistance and Glutathione Peroxidase of Type 2 Diabetic Patients." *Saudi Medical Journal* 32, no. 6 (June 2011): 584–88. PMID: 21666939.

108. Mirtaheri, Elham, Bahram Pourghassem Gargari, Sousan Kolahi, et al. "Effects of Alpha-Lipoic Acid Supplementation on Inflammatory Biomarkers and Matrix Metalloproteinase-3 in Rheumatoid Arthritis Patients." *Journal of the American College of Nutrition* 34, no. 4 (2015): 310–17. doi: 10.1080/07315724.2014.910740.

109. "Lipoic Acid." *Linus Pauling Institute,* April 28, 2014. http://lpi.oregonstate.edu/mic/dietary-factors/lipoic-acid.

110. Ibrahimpasic, Kanita. "Alpha Lipoic Acid and Glycaemic Control in Diabetic Neuropathies at Type 2 Diabetes Treatment." *Medical Archives* 67, no. 1 (2013): 7–9. doi: 10.5455/medarh.2013.67.7-9.

111. Vallianou, Natalia, Angelos Evangelopoulos, and Pavlos Koutalas. "Alpha-Lipoic Acid and Diabetic Neuropathy." *The Review of Diabetic Studies* 6, no. 4 (2009): 230–36. doi: 10.1900/RDS.2009.6.230.

112. "Lipoic Acid." *Linus Pauling Institute,* April 28, 2014. http://lpi.oregonstate.edu/mic/dietary-factors/lipoic-acid.

113. Lazo de la Vega-Monroy, M. L., E. Larrieta, M. S. German, et al. "Effects of Biotin Supplementation in the Diet on Insulin Secretion, Islet Gene Expression, Glucose Homeostasis and Beta-Cell Proportion." *The Journal of Nutritional Biochemistry* 24, no. 1 (January 2013): 169–77. doi: 10.1016/j.jnutbio.2012.03.020.

114. Larrieta, Elena, Maria Luisa Lazo de la Vega-Monroy, Paz Vital, et al. "Effects of Biotin Deficiency on Pancreatic Islet Morphology, Insulin Sensitivity and Glucose Homeostasis." *The Journal of Nutritional Biochemistry* 23, no. 4 (April 2012): 392–99. doi: 10.1016/j.jnutbio.2011.01.003.

115. *Ibid.*

116. Lazo de la Vega-Monroy, M. L., E. Larrieta, M. S. German, et al. "Effects of Biotin Supplementation in the Diet on Insulin Secretion, Islet Gene Expression, Glucose Homeostasis and Beta-Cell Proportion." *The Journal of Nutritional Biochemistry* 24, no. 1 (January 2013): 169–77. doi: 10.1016/j.jnutbio.2012.03.020.

117. *Ibid.*

118. Reddi, A., B. DeAngelis, O. Frank, N. Lasker, and H. Baker. "Biotin Supplementation Improves Glucose and Insulin Tolerances in Genetically Diabetic KK Mice." *Life Sciences* 42, no. 13 (1988): 1323–30. PMID: 3280936.

119. Zhang, Xingwang, Jianping Qi, Yi Lu, et al. "Enhanced Hypoglycemic Effect of Biotin-Modified Liposomes Loading Insulin: Effect of Formulation Variables, Intracellular Trafficking, and Cytotoxicity." *Nanoscale Research Letters* 9, no. 1 (2014): 185. doi: 10.1186/1556-276X-9-185.

120. Fuhr, Joseph P., Hope He, Neil Goldfarb, and David B. Nash. "Use of Chromium Picolinate and Biotin in the Management of Type 2 Diabetes: An Economic Analysis." *Disease Management* 8, no. 4 (August 2005): 265–75. doi: 10.1089/dis.2005.8.265.

121. McCarty, M. F. "High-Dose Biotin, an Inducer of Glucokinase Expression, May Synergize with Chromium Picolinate to Enable a Definitive Nutritional Therapy for Type II Diabetes." *Medical Hypotheses* 52, no. 5 (May 1999): 401–6. doi: 10.1054/mehy.1997.0682.

122. Singer, Gregory M., and Jeff Geohas. "The Effect of Chromium Picolinate and Biotin Supplementation on Glycemic Control in Poorly Controlled Patients with Type 2 Diabetes Mellitus: A Placebo-Controlled, Double-Blinded, Randomized Trial." *Diabetes Technology & Therapeutics* 8, no. 6 (December 2006): 636–43. doi: 10.1089/dia.2006.8.636.

123. Albarracin, Cesar A., Burcham C. Fuqua, Joseph L. Evans, and Ira D. Goldfine. "Chromium Picolinate and Biotin Combination Improves Glucose Metabolism in Treated, Uncontrolled Overweight to Obese Patients with Type 2 Diabetes." *Diabetes/Metabolism Research and Reviews* 24, no. 1 (February 2008): 41–51. doi: 10.1002/dmrr.755.

124. Fuhr, Joseph P., Hope He, Neil Goldfarb, and David B. Nash. "Use of Chromium Picolinate and Biotin in the Management of Type 2 Diabetes: An Economic Analysis." *Disease Management* 8, no. 4 (August 2005): 265–75. doi: 10.1089/dis.2005.8.265.

125. Mudra, Mitchell, Nacide Ercan-Fang, Litao Zhong, et al. "Influence of Mulberry Leaf Extract on the Blood Glucose and Breath Hydrogen Response to Ingestion of 75 G Sucrose by Type 2 Diabetic and Control Subjects." *Diabetes Care* 30, no. 5 (May 1, 2007): 1272–74. doi: 10.2337/dc06-2120.

126. Da Villa, G., G. Ianiro, F. Mangiola, et al. "White Mulberry Supplementation as Adjuvant Treatment of Obesity." *Journal of Biological Regulators and Homeostatic Agents* 28, no. 1 (March 2014): 141–45. doi: 10.1016/S1590-8658(14)60368-6.

127. Knuth, Nicolas D., Darcy L. Johannsen, Robyn A. Tamboli, et al. "Metabolic Adaptation Following Massive Weight Loss Is Related to the Degree of Energy Imbalance and Changes in Circulating Leptin." *Obesity (Silver Spring, Md.)* 22, no. 12 (December 2014): 2563–69. doi: 10.1002/oby.20900.

128. Das, Sai Krupa, Susan B. Roberts, Megan A. McCrory, et al. "Long-Term Changes in Energy Expenditure and Body Composition after Massive Weight Loss Induced by Gastric Bypass Surgery." *The American Journal of Clinical Nutrition* 78, no. 1 (July 2003): 22–30. PMID: 12816767.